Prevention in General Practice

SECOND EDITION

Oxford General Practice Series · 23

Edited by

GODFREY FOWLER

Clinical Reader in General Practice, University of Oxford

MUIR GRAY

Regional Medical Officer, Oxford Regional Health Authority

and

PETER ANDERSON

Former Director, HEA Primary Health Care Unit

OXFORD NEW YORK TOKYO
OXFORD UNIVERSITY PRESS
1993

Oxford University Press, Walton Street, Oxford OX2 6DP
Oxford New York Toronto
Delhi Bombay Calcutta Madras Karachi
Kuala Lumpur Singapore Hong Kong Tokyo
Nairobi Dar es Salaam Cape Town
Melbourne Auckland Madrid
and associated companies in
Berlin Ibadan

Oxford is a trade mark of Oxford University Press

Published in the United States
by Oxford University Press Inc., New York

First published as 'Preventive medicine in general practice' 1985
Second edition 1993

A catalogue record for this book is available from the British Library

Library of Congress Cataloging in Publication Data
(Data available on request)

ISBN 0-19-262158-0

Typeset by Joshua Associates Ltd, Oxford
Printed in Great Britain by
Dotesios Ltd, Trowbridge

OXFORD MEDICAL PUBLICATIONS

Prevention in General Practice

OXFORD GENERAL PRACTICE SERIES

5. Locomotor disability in general practice
   edited by M. I. V. Jayson and R. Million
6. The consultation: an approach to learning and teaching
   D. Pendleton, P. Tate, P. Havelock, and T. Schofield
8. Management in general practice
   P. M. M. Pritchard, K. B. Low, and M. Whalen
9. Modern obstetrics in general practice
   edited by G. N. Marsh
10. Terminal care at home
    edited by R. Spilling
11. Rheumatology for general practitioners
    H. L. F. Currey and S. Hull
12. Women's problems in general practice
    (Second edition)
    edited by Ann McPherson
13. Paediatric problems in general practice
    (Second edition)
    M. Modell and R. H. Boyd
14. Epidemiology in general practice
    edited by D. Morrell
15. Psychological problems in general practice
    A. C. Markus, C. Murray Parkes, P. Tomson, and M. Johnston
16. Research methods for general practitioners
    David Armstrong, Michael Calnan, and John Grace
17. Family problems
    Peter R. Williams
18. Health care for Asians
    B. R. McAvoy
19. Continuing care: the management of chronic disease
    (Second edition)
    edited by J. C. Hasler and T. P. C. Schofield
20. Geriatric problems in general practice
    (Second edition)
    G. K. Wilcock, J. A. M. Gray, and J. M. Longmore
21. Efficient care in general practice
    G. N. Marsh
22. Hospital referrals
    edited by Martin Roland and Angela Coulter
23. Prevention in general practice
    edited by Godfrey Fowler, Muir Gray, and Peter Anderson

Preface

The prevention of disease and the promotion of health are not isolated activities carried out by health professionals. They take place in a context, physical and social, which can have a bearing on the health of individuals and populations as great as, or greater than, the influence of health professionals. Nevertheless, we remain convinced that interaction between health professionals and patients has a vitally important part to play in disease prevention and health promotion.

The outcomes of this interaction may be changes in lifestyle or adoption of measures to reduce risk. However, such outcomes are only one effect of the increasing involvement of primary health care teams in the prevention of disease and promotion of health. Since the first edition of this book, smoking has been discouraged in millions of consultations; it has also become a public health issue. Other ways of preventing disease and promoting health will also have been discussed millions of times. The cumulative effect of all this on individuals, their families, and the communities in which they live is impossible to estimate.

Furthermore, policy changes have been made to encourage general practitioners and other members of primary health care teams to prevent disease and promote health; in particular, the work done by the facilitators for prevention in primary care helped bring about fundamental reappraisal of the part played by what were Family Practitioner Committees and are now Family Health Service Authorities.

The new National Health Service general practice contract has brought about a major shift towards prevention and health promotion in general practice. The basic policy is welcome but some of the details need amendment.

There have been many changes in health care over the past decade, but there has also been continuity. There are still sick people wanting better health as well as healthy people who want to stay healthy or even improve their health. This book has been rewritten completely and retitled in the light of the changes, to assist primary health care teams with their new tasks in prevention. It is concerned with validated and feasible prevention and health promotion. It is intended to be practical but also to include the basic scientific justification for activities recommended. It is mainly concerned with these activities in young and middle-aged adults; other books in this series include contributions on prevention in childhood, adolescence, pregnancy, and old age, so these are not dealt with here.

The book remains aimed at general practitioners—established principals and trainees—but we hope others in primary health care, especially practice nurses who undertake much of the implementation of prevention and health promotion, will find it useful too. Increasing emphasis on this aspect of health care in basic medical education will mean that medical students will find much of it of value also.

Oxford
July 1992

G.F.
M.G.
P.A.

Contents

Contributors

Dr Peter Anderson
HEA Primary Health Care Unit
University Department of Public Health and Primary Care
Churchill Hospital
Oxford OX3 7LJ

Dr Joan Austoker
CRC Primary Care Education Group
University Department of Public Health and Primary Care
65 Banbury Road
Oxford OX2 6PE

Angela Coulter
Health Services Research Unit
University Department of Public Health and Primary Care
Gibson Building
Radcliffe Infirmary
Woodstock Road
Oxford OX2 6HE

Dr Godfrey Fowler
University Department of Public Health and Primary Care
Gibson Building
Radcliffe Infirmary
Oxford
OX2 6HE

Dr Muir Gray
Oxford Regional Health Authority
Old Road
Headington
Oxford OX3 7LF

Gorm Kirsch
Oxford Regional Health Authority
Old Road
Headington
Oxford OX3 7LF

Dr Martin Lawrence
University Department of Public Health and Primary Care
Gibson Building
Radcliffe Infirmary
Oxford OX2 6HE

Dr David Mant
ICRF General Practice Research Group
University Department of Public Health and Primary Care
Gibson Building
Radcliffe Infirmary
Oxford OX2 6HE

Dr Andrew Markus
University Department of Public Health and Primary Health Care
Gibson Building
Radclife Infirmary
Oxford OX2 6HE

Dr Peter Pritchard
31 Martin's Lane
Dorchester on Thames
Oxon OX10 7JF

Dr Theo Schofield
University Department of Public Health and Primary Care
Gibson Building
Radcliffe Infirmary
Oxford OX2 6HE

Dr Richard Mayon-White
Oxfordshire Department of Public Health
Manor House
Headley Way
Oxford OX3 9DZ

Professor Archie Young
Academic Department of Geriatric Medicine
The Royal Free Hospital
London NW3 3QG

1 Health promotion and disease prevention: future challenges

Muir Gray

The emphasis on health promotion and disease prevention has greatly increased in the last decade and these activities are now included in the terms and conditions of service of National Health Service general practitioners in the UK (see the Appendix).

Furthermore, in its recently published consultation document '*The health of the nation*' (1991), the British Government has identified the following challenges:

- Many people still die prematurely or suffer from debilitating ill-health from conditions that are, to a large extent, preventable.
- There are significant variations in health: geographical, social, ethnic, and occupational.
- There are marked variations in the quantity and quality of health care delivered in different parts of the country.

Within the document, objectives and targets for the prevention of ill-health and the promotion of good health are set. Targets for the year 2000 for producing a reduction in the incidences of the major diseases responsible for premature death, and their contributory causes, have been specified (see Chapter 2). Achieving these objectives and targets will depend on a wide variety of activities ranging from changes in individual behaviour to Government actions; but health services, especially primary health services, are identified as having a key part to play.

Population ageing

In all developed countries the number of elderly people is rising; this demographic trend will be the main factor increasing the need for health care, even though other trends will also affect the need for health services, for example, increased smoking among women or the changes taking place in our environment.

It is often thought that an increasing number of older people increases the need for geriatric and psychogeriatric services only, but population ageing affects all health care services (other than paediatrics and obstetrics). For example, a careful analysis of cancer trends carried out by the Health Department in The Netherlands indicated that the number of new cases of cancer would increase by about 1.5 per cent a year, principally due to population ageing. Thus, the number of new cases of cancer will increase by about 15 per cent in the forthcoming decade, largely as a result of an increase in the numbers of elderly people in the population (Cleton and Coebergh 1988).

There is no doubt that AIDS will increase in incidence and prevalence and that this will also increase the demand for health care. However, important though the challenge of AIDS is, it will make less of a demand on resources than population ageing. Furthermore, it does appear that governments are willing to earmark and invest resources for the prevention and management of AIDS, in contrast to the situation relating to the impact of population ageing.

New technology

Although it is impossible to predict the consequences of ongoing and future basic and clinical research, it can be assumed that the number of interventions that will be demonstrated as being effective by well designed and well conducted trials will steadily, perhaps exponentially, increase during the next decade.

The word 'intervention' is used rather than 'technology' because interventions can be classified as 'high technology' or 'low technology'. For example, the demonstration that seven-day home care is effective in maintaining old people in their own homes has led to bids for resources to develop such care.

One definition of a need is that it is a problem for which there is an effective intervention. Using this definition, it can be seen that the need for health care will increase not only as a result of population ageing and the increasing incidence of diseases such as AIDS but also as a result of research and development making new treatments available.

Once more it is important to emphasize that these trends are interrelated. The number of people with cancer at any point in time will increase by about 3 per cent a year. This will occur partly because of the increasing number of new cases, and partly because of earlier detection of disease and longer survival post diagnosis due to the introduction of services such as breast cancer screening, and the development of new, more effective types of care, such as more effective chemotherapeutic agents.

Rising consumerism

In addition to increasing needs, demand will also increase as consumers of health care become not only better educated and informed but also more assertive and better organized. The down-side of this trend is an increased number of complaints and a rising rate of litigation. It is also important to remember, however, that a more-educated population will be better able to understand the complex issues involved in the assessment of risk and effectiveness, and will be better able to appreciate that all health care, including much preventive medicine, consists of balancing risks and benefits—and that there are no quick fixes or golden bullets.

Limited resources

These interrelated challenges will all have to be met within the constraints imposed by limited resources, as shown by the larger outer circle in Fig. 1.1. Resources may be money, skilled staff, or simply the necessary number of young people to provide all the services required, even if money were available. But although it is likely that some increase in resources will occur, and that health workers will continue to campaign and press for more resources for health care, it appears that no government can afford to provide all the resources that will be necessary to meet all of these challenges.

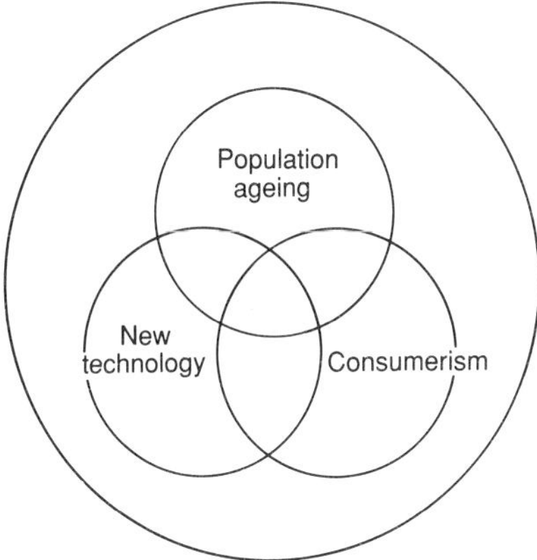

Fig. 1.1 Interrelation between population ageing, new technology, and consumerism. Outer circle represents the constraint imposed by limited resources.

Consequences for health services and primary care teams

These challenges have a number of obvious consequences for all those involved in the provision of health services.

Increasing competition for resources

There will be increasing competition for resources and this competition will become fiercer. It will be essential to demonstrate the efficacy of proposed new interventions or services, preferably by randomized controlled clinical trials, and research in disease prevention or health promotion will have to be rigorously conducted to produce evidence of efficacy. Evidence of efficacy alone will often be insufficient to lead to the introduction of a new service or intervention. Increasingly, those who pay for or 'purchase' health services will expect evidence of effectiveness in ordinary clinical settings as well as the demonstration of efficacy in research studies before investing resources in a new service.

Furthermore, a more critical and sophisticated approach to the assessment of effectiveness will be required, with the need to emphasize more clearly the distinction between absolute and relative risk reduction when describing the benefits of a preventive service. For example, enthusiasts often describe the impact of a preventive service or treatment by describing the relative reduction in risk that will be obtained by prescribing, for example, antihypertensive agents, or drugs to lower cholesterol levels. Those who purchase or pay for health services will want to consider the absolute reduction in risk in a whole population that will be achieved as a result of investing scarce resources in a new service (Brett 1989; Leaf 1989).

Thus there will be a much greater emphasis on cost effectiveness, including the use of measures such as 'quality adjusted life years' (QALYs). This measure discounts a proportion of a year of life according to disability on a scale of 0 (equivalent to death) to 1 (equivalent to full health). One year with 75 per cent disability is 0.25 QALYs i.e. the equivalent of 3 months with full health (Drummond *et al.* 1957). For example, in relation to coronary heart disease prevention, general practitioners' advice to stop smoking is more cost-effective than coronary artery by-pass surgery.

Assessing the appropriateness of health services

In cost-effectiveness studies, the effects of a particular service or intervention are costed. It is then possible to compare the effects that would result from investing resources in a new service with the effects that would be obtained if the same amount of resources were invested in another service, either another preventive service or in some new form of treatment. However, in addition to assessment of costs and benefits the 1990s will see an increasing emphasis on the risks of medical care, and risk–benefit analyses will be carried out in addition to cost–benefit analyses.

The appropriateness of an intervention, either for an individual or for a population, is estimated by considering the costs, risks, and benefits as shown in Fig. 1.2.

A growing concern about the adverse effects of medical care is an inevitable consequence of consumerism. A common cause of patients' complaints is not being informed about the probability of experiencing the side-effects that can be associated with a particular intervention.

It is interesting that the medical profession regards 'effectiveness' as being

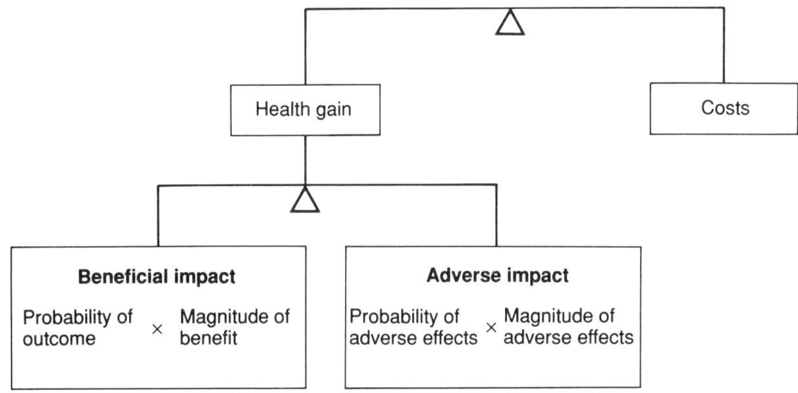

Fig. 1.2 Assessing the appropriateness of an intervention.

synonymous with good effects, but to the consumer adverse effects are just as important as beneficial effects, an issue that became increasingly clear during the 1980s. For example, because of the concern about 'missed' cases of cervical intraepithelial neoplasia, steps were taken to increase the sensitivity of cervical screening by increasing the proportion of women referred for colposcopy. The increase in detection rate from this increase in referral was small, but the increase in adverse effects was great. Every 1 per cent increase in referral results in about 30 000 to 40 000 more women being referred for colposcopy across the country, and being referred for colposcopy has a significant impact on a woman's psychological well-being. Drives to increase the sensitivity of a screening test almost always reduce its specificity with an increasing number of false positives, and false positives almost always have adverse psychological side-effects.

In the 1990s, appraisals of preventive and health promotion activities will have to consider not only the effectiveness but also the appropriateness of the particular intervention being considered. Adequate weighting will have to be given to both the probability and type of side-effect, and the public will expect to be fully informed about the possible adverse effects of interventions or services offered to them.

An increasing emphasis on quality

The effectiveness of a health service is measured by the degree to which it meets its objectives or achieves its outcomes. The quality of a health service is determined by the degree to which it conforms with the standards of care defined for that particular service.

Standards are value judgements, that is levels of achievement arbitrarily chosen and defined in a number of different ways. For a given service, for example, there may be minimum acceptable standards. There may also be achievable standards—the achievability of a standard being defined with respect to actual levels of performance. For example, one way of defining an achievable standard is to measure the level of achievement that can be obtained by three-quarters of primary care teams working in similar conditions; if three-quarters of primary care teams have achieved a certain level of performance it cannot be defined as being 'excellent' or 'optimal'. Excellence is always a worthy goal, but for many primary care teams excellence is unrealistic and it is more helpful to provide an indicator of achievability.

In an imperfect way the national targets for cervical screening are indications of minimum acceptable and achievable standards, although these were set arbitrarily at levels of 50 per cent and 80 per cent, without taking into account differences in socio-economic circumstances in which different practices have to operate.

However imperfect these standards are, they indicate that the public, and therefore the politicians, will expect the profession to set and achieve certain clinical standards. The Department of Health has recently set up a new group primarily concerned with the development of clinical standards.

Disease prevention and health promotion—the social dimension

The 1980s was a decade of the individual, a decade in which social or societal approaches to problems were unfashionable. The focus of political action was on the reassertion of the individual as opposed to the State.

During the 1980s many of the advances in preventive medicine, for example the development of breast cancer screening and the introduction of health checks in primary care, were interventions that focused on the individual. Those who advocated these moves were always clear that the individual and society were interwoven like warp and weft, and that to advocate either social or individual initiatives was to advocate an approach of limited effectiveness. Social changes influence the opinions of individuals and individual actions influence the way in which a society as a whole moves.

References

Brett, A. S. (1989). Treating hypercholesterolaemia. How should practising physicians interpret the data for patients? *New England Journal of Medicine*, **321**, 676–80.

Cleton, F. W. and Coebergh, J. W. W. (1988). Cancer in The Netherlands. Vol. 1. In *Scenarios in cancer 1985–2000*, pp. 137–8. Kluwer, Dordrecht.

Drummond, M. F., Stoddart, G. L., and Torrance, G. W. (1987). *Methods for the economic evaluation of health care programmes.* Oxford University Press.

Leof, A. (1989). Management of hypercholesterolaemia. Are preventive interventions advisable? *New England Journal of Medicine*, **321**, 680–3.

2 Prevention: past and present

Godfrey Fowler

Until registration of births and deaths became compulsory in England and Wales in 1838, there were no reliable figures and it is therefore difficult to be certain about death rates and expectation of life until the middle of the nineteenth century. However, expectation of life for both men and women probably increased by no more than a small amount from prehistoric times until about 1870. There was even periods when expectation of life must have decreased (during the Black Death, for example), and possibly other times when it increased more rapidly than average. But there is evidence that the mortality from certain diseases declined long before any preventive measures were introduced: for example, there were epidemics of typhus in Britain in 1718, 1728, and 1751, each coming after a bad harvest, and the disease then waned as the food supply improved. Leprosy was once common throughout Europe, but disappeared before any effective preventive or curative measures were available, and plague disappeared from Europe for no known reason. Improved food supply may well have been the explanation for this 'prevention' in the past.

But by the latter half of the nineteenth century, population figures were much more reliable, and during this period it is clear there was a dramatic reduction in mortality (see Fig. 2.1). This decline in mortality was due almost entirely to a decrease in deaths from infectious diseases. McKeown (1979) has argued that the decline in tuberculosis mortality accounted for nearly half of the total fall in mortality, a decrease in typhus was responsible for about one-fifth, a decrease in scarlet fever for another fifth, a decrease in cholera, dysentery, and diarrhoea for about one-tenth, and a decline in smallpox for about one-twentieth. Only in the case of smallpox was a preventive measure that focused on the individual important; for the rest of these diseases, the decrease can be attributed to environmental changes that effected the whole community, namely, the provision of clean water, the sanitary disposal of sewage, the provision of better housing, and the general improvement in nutrition.

However, these environmental measures were only the tools of prevention. The underlying reason why the incidence of these diseases declined was that there were several social changes that made the necessary legislation for environmental improvement acceptable to the majority. An important factor was the growth of scientific knowledge in the nineteenth century, although it must be emphasized that the bacterial transmission of disease was not clearly

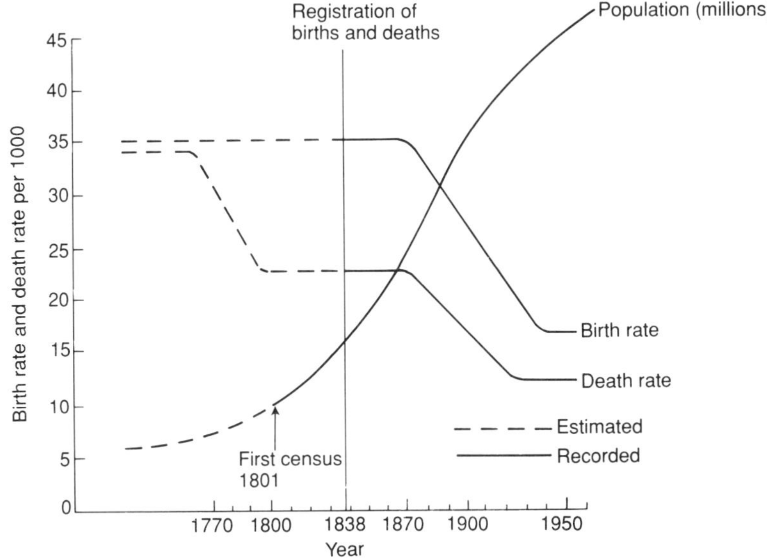

Fig. 2.1 Birth and death rates in the population of England and Wales from 1700 to 1900. (After McKeown and Lowe 1974)

understood until some decades after the most important laws had been passed. There were also many other relevant trends in nineteenth-century society. Philanthropy and paternalism became more important philosophies, the latter fostered to some degree by the need to have a healthy workforce. Poor people became more articulate and the rich became very afraid of some of the diseases, particularly of cholera, which spread due to the insalubrious conditions of nineteenth-century cities. Finally, Britain became wealthy enough to implement the changes that Parliament had deemed necessary.

Prevention in the nineteenth century was therefore largely mediated by government action through legislation, and this legislation improved the quality of life of the majority of people, who enjoyed clean, safe water, better working conditions, and freedom from offensive smells and other 'nuisances'. That is not to say that there was no opposition to preventive medicine in the nineteenth century. On the contrary, there was vociferous and vehement opposition both to vaccination and to environmental improvement, not so much because of the measures involved (which were in themselves generally welcomed) but because they were imposed by law and because they increased the power of central Government.

In developed countries in the twentieth century, the causes of death and disease, and therefore the scope for health improvement are different. But the means for achieving health improvement have many similarities and require Government as well as individual action. Both the provision of preventive services and social changes are necessary for disease prevention and health promotion to be effective, particularly in the poorest groups in society (see Chapter 3).

The scope for prevention today

A major factor which has influenced acknowledgment of the scope for prevention in the late twentieth century has been the growth in and increasing recognition of the importance of epidemiology. This has demonstrated—with varying degrees of certainty—the causes of much of the morbidity and premature mortality at the present time. In Britain and other developed countries the diseases of the past (and many of those of the present in developing countries) related to infections and undernutrition. These have been replaced in developed countries, and are rapidly being replaced in the developing ones, by the 'diseases of affluence' (see Fig. 2.2). The major killers today are diseases of the circulatory system (chiefly, heart attacks and strokes) and cancer. Individual behaviour contributes substantially to these, but the social environment also plays an important part. Overeating and unhealthy nutrition, cigarette smoking, and alcohol consumption contribute substantially, accidents and suicides are important causes of death in early life, and HIV/AIDS demonstrates that, like syphilis in the past, sexually transmitted disease can be devastating.

Persuading and helping people to lead healthy lifestyles is the major challenge for prevention at the present time and the new general practice contract (see the Appendix), which was introduced into the National Health Service in the UK in 1990, acknowledges this by requiring general practitioners to introduce lifestyle enquiry and advice into their everyday practice.

The scope for prevention can be listed under broad headings (see Box 2.1).

Box 2.1: The scope for prevention

Socio-economic improvements
Modification of personal habits
Protection against trauma
Control of infection
Control of pollution
Screening
Prophylactic medication

There is particular scope for the prevention of premature deaths. Taking an arbitrary 'cut-off' of 65 years, as being the common age of retirement,

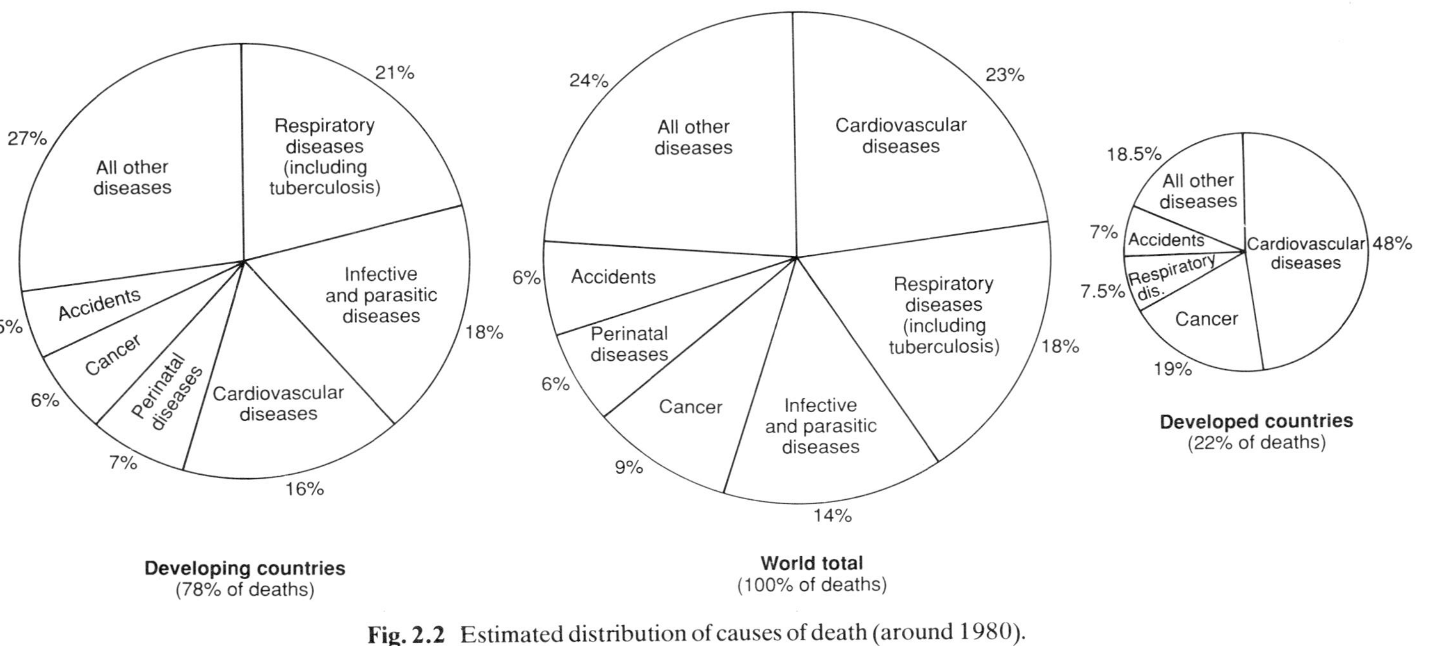

Fig. 2.2 Estimated distribution of causes of death (around 1980).

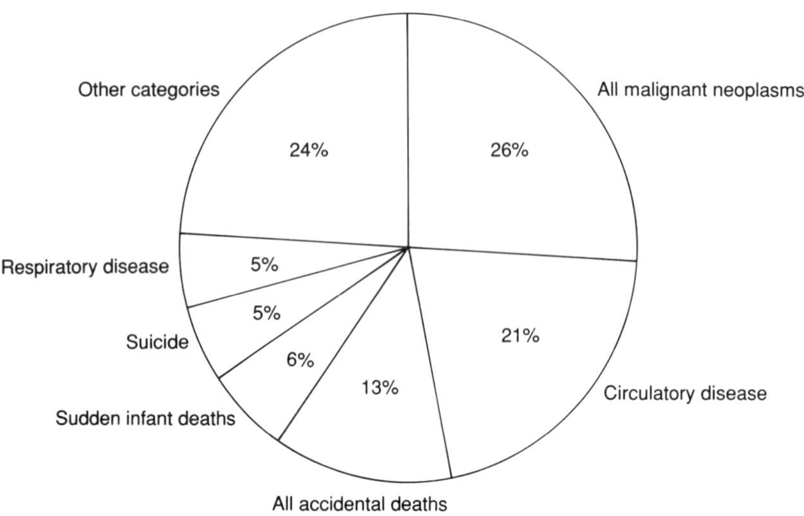

Fig. 2.3 Distribution of years of life lost up to age 65 years (excluding deaths under 28 days) by cause of death for England and Wales (all persons, 1988).

years of 'life lost' by those dying before this age provides a particularly significant measure of the potential gain from prevention. Distribution of total years of life lost by those dying before the age of 65 is illustrated in Fig. 2.3.

As in the past, socio-economic factors continue to play a very important part in health and their influence was highlighted by the *Black report* (Townsend *et al.* 1988). Mortality rates in the lowest socio-economic group are about double those in the highest group, and the gap seems to be widening. Although mortality from all causes has been declining in recent years in all social classes, the decline has been steeper in the upper socio-economic groups and, in women, death rates from coronary heart disease and lung cancer have actually increased in those in lower socio-economic groups. The influence of socio-economic factors on health is discussed in detail in Chapter 3.

Modification of personal habits is a vital part of prevention today and individual chapters in this book discuss smoking (Chapter 9), eating (Chapter 10), alcohol (Chapter 11), stress (Chapter 12), and exercise (Chapter 13). The scope for prevention of morbidity and premature death by attention to these lifestyle issues is considerable. Unhealthy diets, tobacco smoking, and a lack of exercise are major contributors to cardiovascular disease which accounts for almost half of all deaths. Coronary heart disease is the single most important killer in Britain and other developed countries, and has particular importance as a cause of almost half of all deaths in middle-aged men. Encouragingly, in many countries coronary heart disease mortality has been

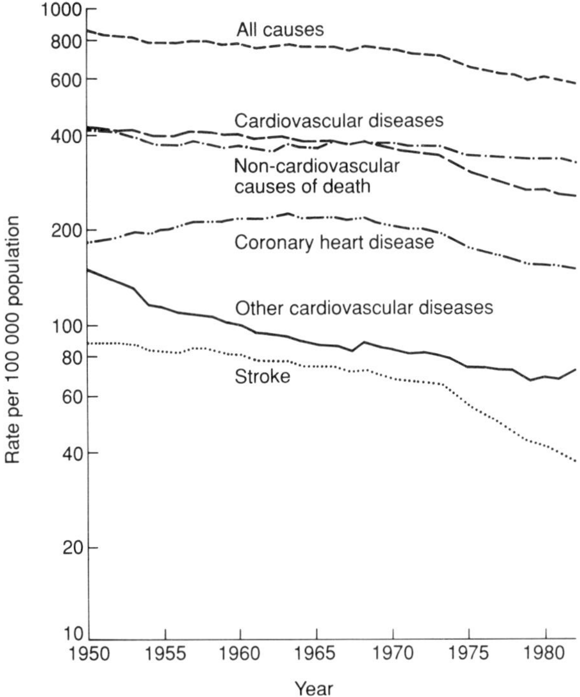

Fig. 2.4 Death rates 1950–1982 for all causes of death, all cardiovascular causes and subgroups, and all non-cardiovascular causes.

declining steeply in recent years. In Britain too coronary heart disease mortality is now declining and stroke mortality has been falling for many years (see Fig. 2.4).

As well as being a major contributor to cardiovascular disease, tobacco smoking is also responsible for about one-third of all cancer deaths. Elimination of this habit would therefore have a major impact on cardiovascular disease, on cancer (especially lung cancer), and on respiratory diseases. In reviewing the evidence for the preventality of cancer, Doll and Peto (1982) emphasized the importance of tobacco—and also the probable importance of dietary factors, though the evidence here is established with less certainty (see Table 2.1).

While the evidence relating tobacco smoking to disease is conclusive, there are still some uncertainties about the modifications of diet which are necessary to a healthy lifestyle, though even here the evidence is becoming steadily more certain. It seems likely that that not only is the risk of cardiovascular disease reduced by a diet low in saturated fats and containing high proportions of fruit, vegetables, and wholegrain cereals but the cancer risk may

Table 2.1 Proportions of cancer deaths attributed to various different factors. (From Doll and Peto 1982.)

Factor or class of factors	Per cent of all cancer deaths	
	Best estimate	Range of acceptable estimates
Tobacco	30	25–40
Alcohol	3	2–4
Diet	35	10–70
Food additives	<1	−5*–2
Reproductive and sexual behaviour	7	1–13
Occupation	4	2–8
Pollution	2	<1–5
Industrial products	<1	<1–2
Medicines and medical procedures	1	0.5–3
Geophysical factors	3	2–4
Infection	10?	1–?
Unknown	?	?

*Allowing for a possibly protective effect of antioxidants and other preservatives.

be reduced too. Such a diet will also facilitate the avoidance of obesity which is so widespread.

Trauma accounts for about 15 000 accidental deaths a year—about 3 per cent of total deaths. But although relatively small in number these deaths assume particular importance in terms of preventive potential because of the relative youth of many of the victims. About one-third of these accidental deaths occur in road traffic accidents but, encouragingly, in spite of the steady growth in the numbers of motor vehicles, road traffic deaths are falling, a favourable trend which is partly attributable to the effects of legislation in the shape of drinking and driving and seatbelt laws. Wearing seatbelts reduces risk of injury by about one-quarter and of death by almost two-thirds. Sadly, in spite of the drink-driving law in Britain, with its legal limit of 80 mg per 100 ml of blood, it is estimated that at least a quarter of all road traffic deaths (and a higher proportion in young men) are associated with alcohol use.

Control of infection was the most successful method of prevention in the past. This control was achieved initially by preventing the spread of the infectious agent, and subsequently methods of immunization against infections were introduced. As a method of protection against infection, immunization is today taken very much for granted, so much so that there is a risk of complacency with consequent failure to achieve population coverage even for such infectious diseases as were a recent scourge and can now be controlled, as, for example, whooping cough and measles. Much current interest in vaccines centres on the possibility of protecting against HIV infection.

As has been discussed much prevention at the present time relates to lifestyle issues which may be seen as primarily a matter for individuals and society rather than health professionals. But one aspect of prevention in which health professionals need to play a central role is screening. This issue is considered in detail in Chapter 8 which describes the potential for and limits of screening procedures in the adult population. Suffice it therefore to say here that all screening procedures warrant a cautious approach and that it is essential that ethical and scientific criteria are satisfied, and that the workload implications are acknowledged and met before screening is undertaken.

Prevention of morbidity

Some criticize preventive medicine because they believe it simply postpones death and increases the number of disabled, elderly people. But the evidence suggests that, although prevention (or treatment) may increase life expectancy, it does not increase the biological lifespan; a higher proportion of people avoid premature deaths and survive to die at an older age. This can be expressed diagrammatically as a change in the shape of the curve relating deaths to age; this becomes a taller, narrower, and more symmetrical with a peak nearer to four-score years than three-score years and ten (see Fig. 2.5).

An alternative way of illustrating this is by the use of survival curves which plot the percentage of a cohort surviving at each age. Reduction in the proportion of premature deaths results in 'rectangularization' of the survival curve as illustrated in Fig. 2.6.

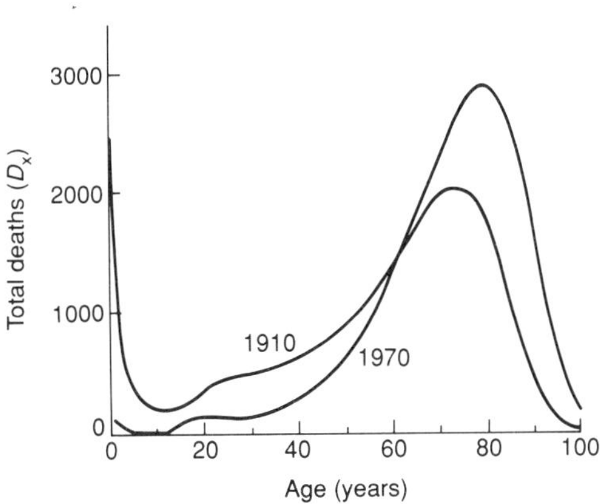

Fig. 2.5 Total deaths per year against age (for the United States, 1910 and 1970). There is a decrease in early deaths with a corresponding increase in late deaths in 1970 as compared with 1910. (From Fries and Crapo 1981)

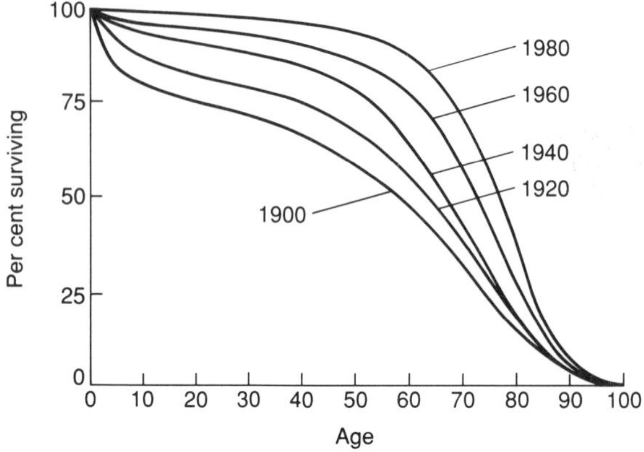

Fig. 2.6 Human survival curves for 1900, 1920, 1940, 1960, and 1980. The curves converge at the same maximum age, thereby demonstrating that the maximum age of survival has been fixed over this period of observation. (From Fries and Crapo 1981)

Moreover, preventive medicine does not simply prevent premature deaths due to disease; by preventing the diseases themselves, it also prevents disability. The effect is not only to postpone the onset of disablement, but to shorten the period of terminal disability and dependency—to 'die young as late as possible'.

The health of the nation

In 1991, the UK Government published a consultative document '*The health of the nation*' which sets out a strategy for improving and protecting the health of the population. It identifies objectives and targets which concern Government, health professionals, and the public.

The major theme of the document is the prevention of ill-health and the promotion of good health and it emphasizes its need to find the right balance between prevention, treatment and rehabilitation. Changes in behaviour—in relation to smoking, alcohol consumption, diet, exercise, avoidance of accidents, and avoidance of sexually transmitted diseases—are seen as important. Both the exercise of individual responsibility and government action are seen as necessary—the latter in provision of information and, where necessary, regulation and legislation.

Key areas where improvements can be made are suggested:

1. Causes of substantial mortality:
   - coronary heart disease;
   - stroke;

- cancers;
- accidents.

2. Causes of substantial ill-health:
   - mental health;
   - diabetes;
   - asthma.
3. Factors which contribute to mortality, ill-health, and healthy living;
   - smoking;
   - diet and alcohol;
   - physical exercise.
4. Areas where there is clear scope for improvement;
   - health of pregnant women, infants, and children;
   - rehabilitation services for people with physical disability;
   - environmental quality.
5. Area where there is great potential for harm:
   - HIV/AIDS;
   - other communicable disease;
   - food safety.

Targets are proposed and these include:

1. For coronary heart disease:
   - 30 per cent reduction nationally in death below age 65 between 1988 and 2000;
   - targets for treatment (e.g. coronary artery bypass surgery and for thrombolytic therapy).
2. For stroke:
   - 30 per cent reduction nationally in death below 65 between 1988 and 2000;
   - 25 per cent reduction nationally in death in the 65–74-year age-group between 1988 and 2000;
   - targets for stroke incidence, early detection and treatment of raised blood pressure, and rehabilitation of stroke survivors.
3. For cancer:
   - 25 per cent reduction nationally in breast cancer deaths in those invited for screening by 2000 compared with 1990;
   - ensure that all women in the eligible age-group have been invited for cervical cancer screening by the end of 1993.
4. For smoking:
   - reduction proportion of men smoking cigarettes from 33 per cent to 22 per cent and of women from 30 per cent to 21 per cent by 2000.
5. For eating and drinking habits:
   - increase the proportion of people deriving less than 15 per cent of their energy from *saturated* fats to at least 60 per cent by 2005;

- increase the proportion of people deriving less than 35 per cent of their food energy from *total* fat to at least 50 per cent by 2005;
- reduce proportion of obese (BMI>30) adults to less than 7 per cent by 2005;
- reduce proportion of those drinking more than sensible limits to less than 1 in 6 men and 1 in 18 women by 2005.

Implementation of this strategy depends on a very broad range of approaches and activities involving the whole spectrum of organizations and individuals from government to ordinary individuals. Health professionals, especially those in primary care, have a key role to play, but it is important that the acknowledgement of their crucial importance does not imply they should be allowed to become overburdened.

References and further reading

Cipolla, C. M. (1962). *The economic history of world population*. Penguin, London.

Doll, R. and Peto, R. (1982). *The causes of cancer*. Oxford University Press.

Fries, J. F. and Crapo, L. M. (1981). *Vitality and ageing: implications of the rectangular curve*. Freeman, San Francisco.

Gray, J. A. M. (1979). *Man against disease*. Oxford University Press.

Marmot, M. G. and McDowell, M. E. (1986). Mortality decline and widening social inequalities. *The Lancet* **ii**, 274–6.

McKeown, K. (1979). *The role of medicine: dream, mirage or nemesis?* Blackwell, Oxford.

McKeown, T. and Lowe, C. R. (1974). *An introduction to social medicine*. Blackwell, Oxford.

McNeill, W. H. (1976). *Plagues and people*. Penguin, London.

Secretary of State for Health (1991). The health of the nation. HMSO, London.

Townsend, P., Davidson, N., and Whitehead, M. (ed.) (1988). *Inequalities in health: the Black Report and health divide*. Penguin, London.

3 Socio-economic influences on health

Angela Coulter

Inequalities in death rates

Social class inequalities in health constitute one of the most fundamental problems in British social policy. Men and women in the lowest social classes run twice the risk of premature death as those in the professional groups. Social class differences in standardized mortality ratios (SMR) are apparent for both sexes from birth to retirement age (Fig. 3.1). A child born to parents who are unskilled workers is twice as likely to die in the first year of life as the child of professional families.

The social class differences are even more dramatic when deaths from specific causes are considered:

- Working class men are twice as likely to die of coronary heart disease and three times more likely to die of lung cancer, than men in middle class occupations.
- Women in social class V run three times the risk of dying from cancer of the cervix, when compared with social class I women.
- Children of social class V parents are four times more likely to die as a result of accidents in and outside the home, than are children of social class I parents.

A recent review of the evidence conducted by an independent multi-disciplinary committee chaired by Professor Alwyn Smith, '*The nation's health*', calculated that if manual workers had sustained the same death rates as non-manual workers in 1981, there would be 42 000 fewer deaths each year in the age-range 16–74 years. In a graphic illustration of the scale of the problem, they pointed out that the total excess mortality for all age-groups in the manual classes amounts to the equivalent of a major air crash or ship-wreck every day of the year.

Inequalities in disease

Social class gradients are also apparent for many common and non-life-threatening illnesses.

In a nationwide survey of a random sample of over 9000 British adults

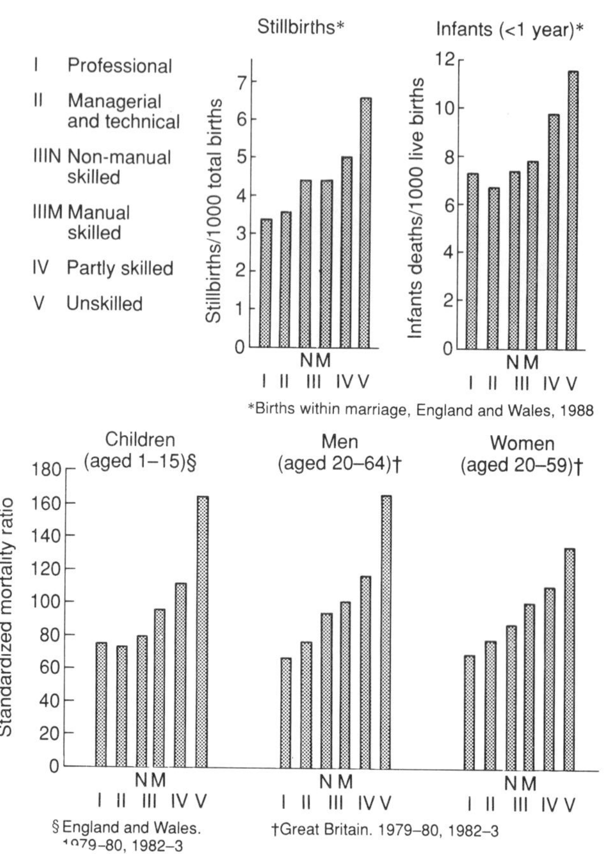

Fig. 3.1 Social class and mortality in Britain. (Source: Delamotte 1991)

conducted in 1984–5, people were asked about symptoms experienced during the four weeks prior to the survey. Women reported more symptoms than men, and in the 40–59 year age-group women in the lowest income group reported nearly twice as many symptoms as those in the highest group. Among men there were threefold differences in illness scores between those with high and low incomes. These differences persisted among those over 60 years.

In the same survey, an increased prevalence of hypertension was found among women in the manual groups and there was a pronounced social class trend in poor respiratory function, which was more common among men and women in the lowest social classes. Similar social class gradients were found for psychological symptoms, such as depression and neuroticism.

Increasing inequalities

Despite the continuing fall in overall death rates, social class inequalities have been widening in Britain since the 1950s. Prior to this period, death rates from some major causes, for example cancer of the lung, were fairly similar across the social classes; since that time the reduction in risk of death from this disease has occurred at a much faster rate among people in the highest social groups (Fig. 3.2).

Comparisons of social class inequalities over time are difficult to evaluate because of changes in the occupational structure of the population. However, there is now convincing evidence that inequalities between manual and

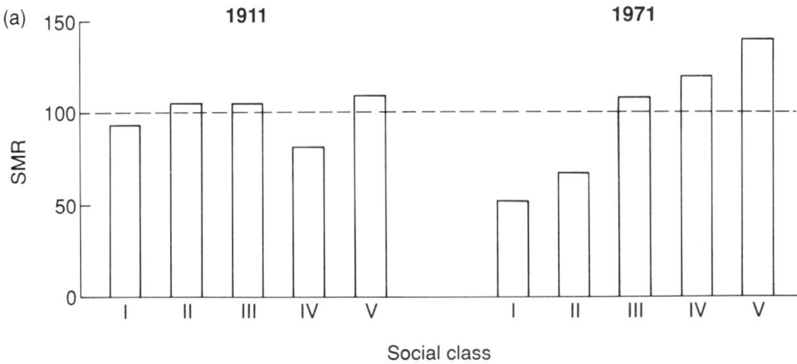

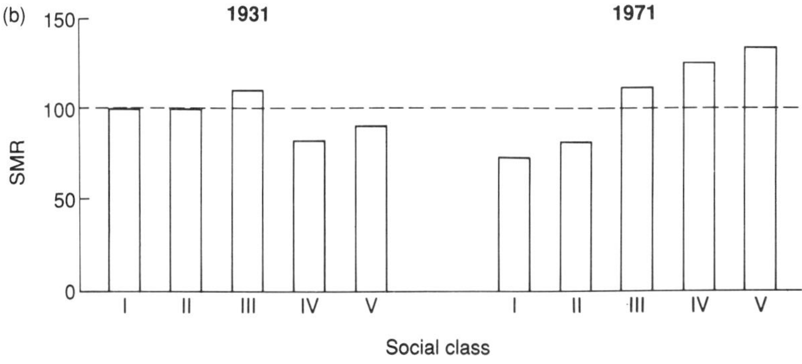

Fig. 3.2 Lung cancer SMRs. (a) Men aged 20–64 (1911) and 15–64 (1971) by social class. (b) Married women at ages 35-64 (1931) and 15–64 (1971). (From Logan 1982)

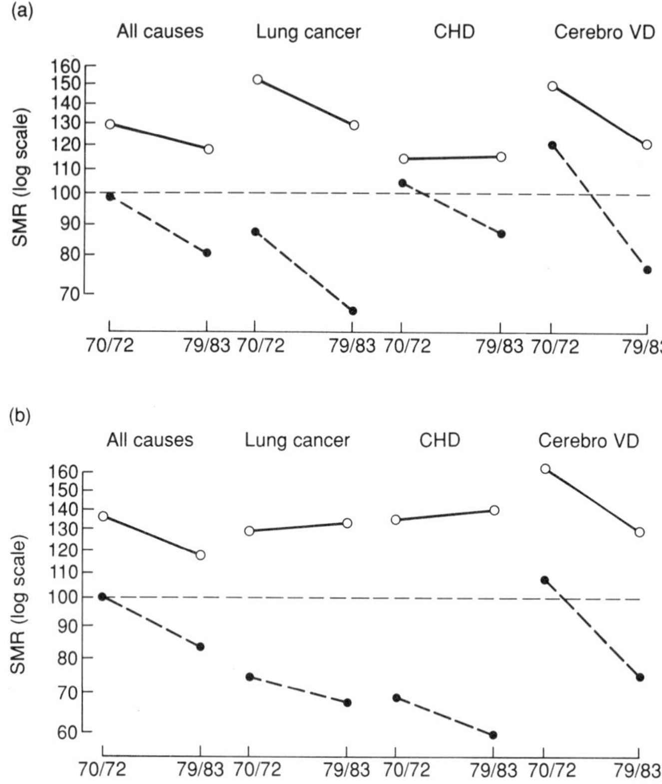

Fig. 3.3 Standardized mortality ratios (SMR) for selected causes of death in Great Britain 1970–2 and 1979–83 for manual (open circles) and non-manual (full circles) groups. (a) Men aged 20–64. (b) Married women aged 20–54 classified by husband's occupation. (For each cause the SMR in 1979–83 is 100 for each sex.) (From Marmot and McDowell 1986)

non-manual groups have persisted, and indeed widened, in the years between 1970 and 1983 (Fig. 3.3).

Regional inequalities

These social class inequalities in the risk of disease and death persist in all parts of the United Kingdom, and they are also apparent in many other Western developed countries. However, within Britain there are also regional differences that cannot be explained wholly in terms of the class structure of the different parts of the country.

In a study (Townsend *et al.* 1988) examining the relationship between health and deprivation, it was found that age-standardized death rates were 31 per cent higher in the north of England than in the south east. People in working class occupations living in prosperous areas—and even in relatively well-off wards within the most deprived region—experienced better health than those of a similar social class living in areas characterized by multiple deprivation. Low income, unstable employment, and poor housing were strongly associated with the geographical differences in the health status of the population.

Unemployment and ill-health

The relationship between unemployment and ill-health has been the subject of much debate, since it is very difficult to determine the extent to which unemployment is a cause of ill-health, or whether people with a prior disposition to ill-health are more likely to be made redundant or to face difficulty in finding a new job. Nevertheless it is now fairly well established that unemployed people do suffer worse health than people in paid employment. They experience higher mortality rates, more chronic illness, more psychological distress, and are more likely to attempt suicide. Even the threat of redundancy can produce an increase in illness and general practice consultations.

The stress of unemployment or threatened unemployment and the associated financial problems has been shown to affect the health of the wives and children of unemployed men. There is also evidence that women who do not have a paid job experience more ill-health than women who work outside the home, and couples where both partners are out of work suffer the greatest levels of stress and ill-health.

Ethnicity and health

There is very little information on the health of British-born members of ethnic minority groups, but the infant mortality rate is known to be higher than the UK average for babies born to mothers from the West Indies and the Indian subcontinent. First-generation immigrants of Asian origin have been found to be at greater risk of mortality from coronary heart disease, despite their lower prevalence of smoking and heavy drinking. They are also more likely to have non-insulin-dependent diabetes and much more likely to suffer from tuberculosis.

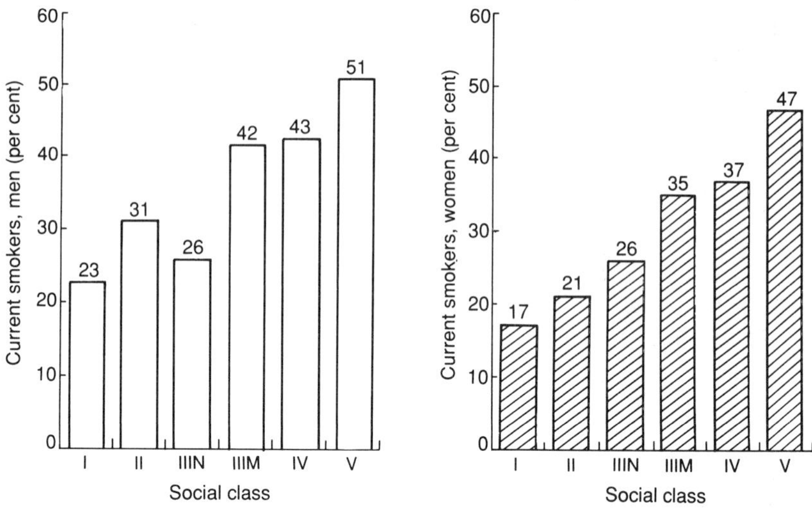

Fig. 3.4 Incidence of smoking by social class. (Source: Healthy Life Survey, Oxford Region 1988)

Social class differences in lifestyles

Part of the explanation for these differences in the risk of ill health lies in the differences between the groups in 'unhealthy' or risk-taking behaviour. Between 1985 and 1988 a random population survey of over 11 000 adults was undertaken in the Oxford region (which includes the counties of Oxfordshire, Buckinghamshire, Berkshire, and Northamptonshire), with the aim of collecting information about health-related behaviour among the different sections of the community. The results illustrate considerable social class differences in the lifestyles of people in this relatively prosperous part of the country.

Smoking

Men and women in social class V were more than twice as likely to be smokers as men and women in social class I (Fig. 3.4). When these results are adjusted to take account of age differences between the groups, the difference between the top and bottom social classes rises to threefold for the men and nearly fourfold among the women.

Men and women who were unemployed were more likely to be smokers than those in paid employment, especially if their partner was also unemployed.

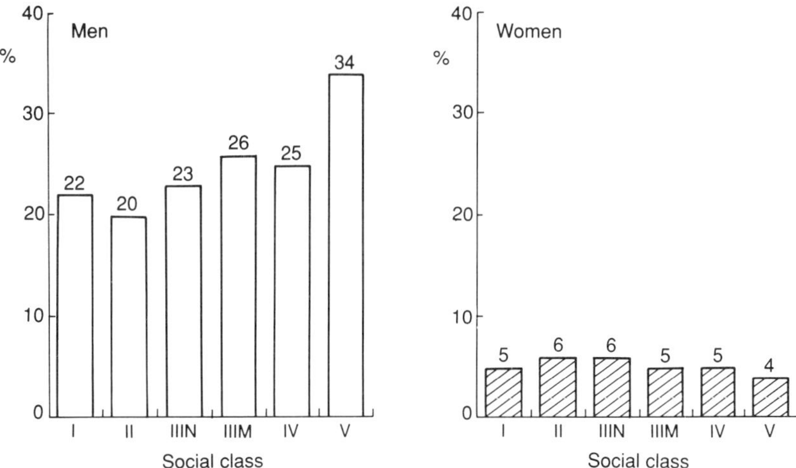

Fig. 3.5 Alcohol consumption by social class (per cent consuming more than the recommended limit for their sex). (Source: Healthy Life Survey, Oxford Region 1988)

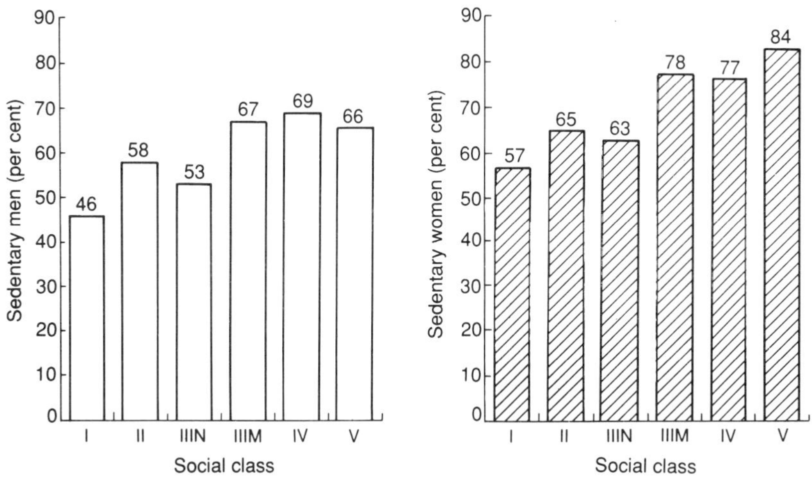

Fig. 3.6 Sedentary lifestyles by social class. (Source: Healthy Life Survey, Oxford Region 1988)

Alcohol consumption

Very few women reported high levels of alcohol consumption, despite the fact that the recommended limit is lower for women than for men (Fig. 3.5). Men in social class V were more likely to drink more than the sensible recommended limit (21 standard units per week) than those in the other groups, but among women alcohol consumption was not related to social class.

Unemployed men were no more likely to drink heavily than those in paid employment.

Alcohol consumption was highest among young men.

Exercise

In this survey a sedentary lifestyle was defined as one in which participation in vigorous sport or recreational activities occurred less than once a month. This again was strongly related to social class, with those in the lower social classes reporting less recreational exercise than those in the higher groups (Fig. 3.6). However, if work-related exercise is taken into account, the gradient is reversed among the men due to the greater participation in manual labour among those in social classes IIIM, IV, and V, but not amongst the women.

Diet

Dietary patterns were strongly related to social class. An 'unhealthy' diet was defined as one in which the foods consumed were high in saturated fat, low in fibre, and high in sugar. After adjustment for age, working class men were found to be almost four times more likely to report unhealthy diets as men in social class I and there was more than a sixfold difference between social class I and social class V women (Fig. 3.7).

People in working class occupations were much less likely to eat wholemeal bread, polyunsaturated fats, skimmed milk, and fresh fruit and vegetables, and much more likely to consume less healthy food such as processed meats, cakes and biscuits, white bread, and full-fat milk.

Weight

A body mass index (weight in kilograms over height in metres, squared) of not more than 25 for males or 24 for females was taken as the standard for acceptable healthy weight. The prevalence of overweight was, like smoking, diet, and exercise, strongly associated with social class among women (Fig. 3.8).

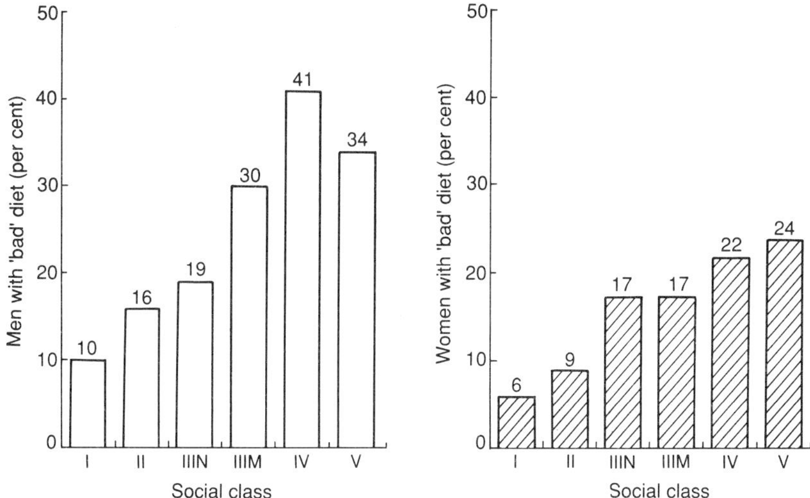

Fig. 3.7 Incidence of 'unhealthy diets' by social class. (Source: Healthy Life Survey, Oxford Region 1988)

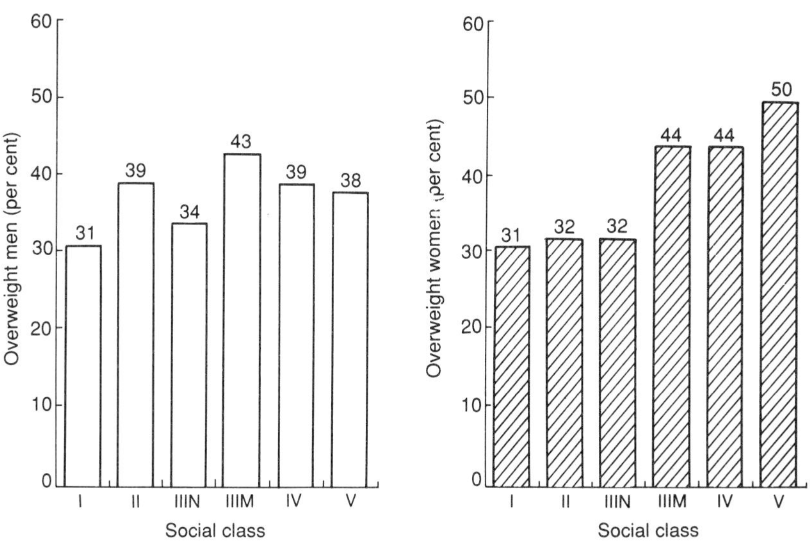

Fig. 3.8 Overweight by social class. (Source: Healthy Life Survey, Oxford Region 1988)

Cervical screening

The Oxford survey also provided evidence of inequalities in the utilization of routine screening procedures. The number of women who reported having a cervical smear varied by age and social class (Table 3.1), with those known to be at greatest risk of developing cervical cancer, i.e. older working class women, being the least likely to have had an up-to-date screening test.

Table 3.1 Proportions of women (as a percentage) reporting a cervical smear test within the last five years (by age and social class)†

Social class	Age				
	18–24	25–34	35–44	45–54	55–64
I	89	89	90	78	64
II	71	93	90	75	60
IIIN	59	82	87	88	58
IIIM	79	90	84	73	55
IV	58	84	81	68	45
V	72	70	73	61	55

†All women: not adjusted for hysterectomy status. (Source: Healthy Life Survey, Oxford Region, 1988)

Blood pressure screening

Blood pressure measurement also varied by sex and social class (Fig. 3.9) and again there was evidence that some people in high-risk groups were not being regularly screened, particularly among the men.

Other factors

Although these lifestyle differences can account for some of the socio-economic differences in health status and risk of premature death, they cannot account for it all. It is likely that a variety of other factors, the effects of which are more difficult to measure, influence the poorer health experience of people in the less advantaged groups (see Box 3.1).

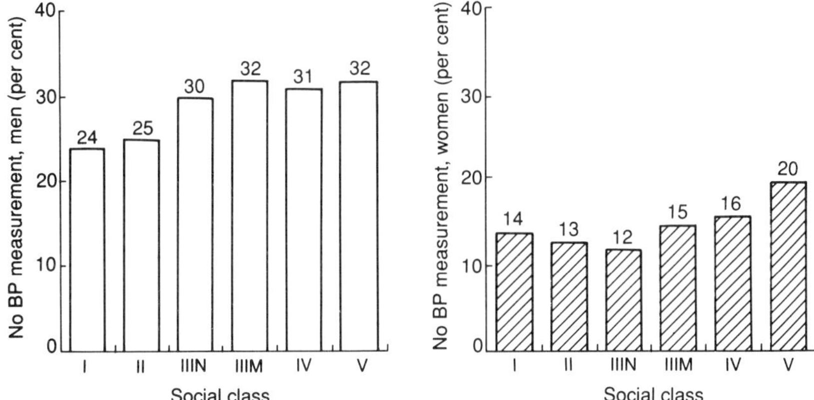

Fig. 3.9 Percentage of men and women who have had no blood pressure measurement within the last five years, by social class. (Source: Healthy Life Survey, Oxford Region 1988)

Implications for primary care

If primary health care teams are to make any impact on the prevention of avoidable mortality and morbidity, it will be necessary to devise strategies for tackling the inequalities described above. There are three essential planks to such a strategy: understanding, targeting, and advocacy.

Understanding behaviour

If the promotion of healthier lifestyles is to be successful it must be based on an understanding of why people behave as they do. The factors affecting the decision to smoke or drink or to eat unhealthy food are very complex and simplistic explanations are almost always wrong.

For example, the assumption that people smoke simply because they are ignorant of the risks is no longer tenable. Although many people are vague about the details and magnitude of the risks, survey after survey has shown that most people in all social classes know that smoking is harmful.

Interviews with people living in stressful situations, such as Hilary Graham's study of working class mothers of young children living in relative poverty (Graham 1984), have found that they often rationalize their smoking habit in terms of the short-term benefits to be gained. Smoking can provide the only relief and relaxation in an otherwise stressful existence. Telling these women that they may die from lung cancer, or that passive smoking may

Box 3.1: Factors other than lifestyle adversely influencing health

- Low income, which affects the extent to which people are in a position to make lifestyle choices.
- Occupationally related stress, which may have a more adverse effect on those who are not in a position to control the pace at which they work.
- The threat of unemployment.
- Occupational hazards.
- Pollution, at work and in the home environment.
- Lack of social support from families and friends.
- Poor housing, especially if it is damp and/or overcrowded.
- Lack of recreational amenities.
- Lack of transport.
- Lack of time and/or space for relaxation.
- Social pressures, e.g. to smoke, drink to excess, or to eat an unhealthy diet.
- Commercial pressures, to smoke, drink, and eat unhealthy food.
- Inadequate education, including the failure to teach about the determinants of health.
- The failure on the part of health administrators and health professionals to tailor their services to meet the needs of less-advantaged people.

harm their children, without helping them in other ways, may only add to their burdens.

Nevertheless, there is plenty of evidence of a desire among members of all social groups to adopt a healthier lifestyle. There is also evidence that people now expect to receive health and lifestyle advice from their general practitioners.

In designing a strategy to put prevention into practice, members of primary health care teams should take account of the guidelines shown in Box 3.2.

Targeting: the population approach

Tackling social class inequalities in health risks in a general practice setting requires a shift from a reactive to a proactive approach. The essential philosophical change is from the traditional view of the registered patients as a collection of individuals, whose needs are dealt with as and when they decide to consult with a specific health problem, to seeing the practice as a

Box 3.2: Guidelines for designing a strategy to implement prevention

- Everyone lives in a social world and faces many competing social pressures. Advice which ignores this and focuses only on the individual is unlikely to be effective. Blaming the victim is no way to achieve change.
- Lay beliefs about health and illness are often complex and sophisticated, although they may differ from those of health professionals. An effective health promotion strategy should start by looking at the problem from the perspective of the people at whom it is aimed.
- Studies have shown that general practitioners are better at communicating with middle class patients, whose consultation times tend to be longer and to whom they are much more likely to give detailed explanations. It is important not to assume that working class people do not want or cannot absorb information relating to their health. Everyone has a right to full and honest information about matters of such crucial personal concern.
- What is required is a sensitive approach to giving health advice in primary care which recognizes the social constraints which affect people's behaviour, and the different 'opportunity costs' faced by people in different socio-economic groups.
- A healthy diet may be relatively expensive for those on low incomes, or difficult to prepare for those with inadequate facilities or a limited choice of shops. Effective advice should extend to helping people to devise strategies for overcoming these problems.
- Advice on cessation of smoking and reduction of alcohol consumption should start from an understanding of the reasons why people smoke and drink, and the social context in which they do it. It may be appropriate to suggest alternative strategies for coping with stress.
- Recreation facilities are not as accessible to those without transport or to those with small chilren, and they may be expensive. Practical advice could suggest ways of incorporating greater levels of healthy exercise into normal daily life.
- Assistance with finding child-care facilities or help with the care of elderly dependants, or advice about social security benefits or housing problems, may in the long run achieve more than simple exhortations to reduce risk factors.

Box 3.3: Elements of a proactive approach to promoting health

- Screening, i.e. offering appointments at preventive care clinics to specific groups, for example all people in a particular age-group. Non-attenders can be followed up, either at their next visit to the surgery, or if necessary with a home visit.
- Keeping accurate records and registers. These should include details such as occupation, employment, and marital status and should be regularly updated. Risk factors and attendance at preventive clinics should also be recorded. The record system should be designed to facilitate easy retrieval of information, and computers offer tremendous advantages in this regard.
- Audit and monitoring. The extent to which coverage of the whole population is being achieved should be regularly monitored. Once the practice team becomes aware of the gaps in coverage, the next task is to investigate the reasons and to devise strategies to overcome any weaknesses in the system. This may involve targeting specific groups for particular attention.

population, with the primary health care team playing an important part in promoting the health of the whole population.

Elements of a proactive approach are shown in Box 3.3.

There is some evidence that opportunistic screening programmes fail to reach those most at risk (Waller *et al.* 1980). One practice, which was concerned about the low uptake of preventive services among the more deprived members of their practice population, devised a successful strategy for tackling the problem (Marsh and Channing 1988). Their plan of action is described in Box 3.4.

Advocacy and the public health approach

Although, as we have seen, there is plenty of scope for tackling inequalities in health in a general practice setting, there are also limits to what can be achieved. Unless we move towards creating the conditions which make it easier for people in all social classes to make healthy choices, there is a danger that, despite all the best efforts of primary health care teams, the gap will continue to widen.

What is needed is a comprehensive public health approach, involving the community and the coordinated efforts of health authorities and central government. This would involve thinking about the health implications of the

Box 3.4: Marsh and Channing's strategy for increasing the uptake of preventive services among deprived members of the practice population

1. First they made a systematic study of their practice records, comparing groups of 'deprived' patients from a local authority housing estate within the area, with an 'endowed' group matched for age and sex, living in a pleasant private housing estate in another part of the practice.

2. They found that the deprived patients had:
- more serious physical illness;
- more hospital admissions;
- more casualty attendances;
- more mental illness;
- more referrals to consultants;
- more GP consultations;
- fewer childhood immunizations;
- more teenage pregnancies;
- more pregnancies terminated;
- fewer cervical smears among older women;
- lower attendance for preventive health checks;
- more smokers.

3. They decided that their existing system of 'fairly informal extra effort—health visitors spending more time in the area, paying opportunistic attention to the deprived families when they presented, and the presence of a small peripheral community clinic operated by the district health authority'—was failing to provide adequate preventive care for the deprived community.

4. They therefore adopted an intensive programme aimed at the deprived group, which included the following elements:
   - A prevention card covering smoking status, tetanus immunization, blood pressure measurement, urine tests, attendance at well-man and well-woman clinics, family planning advice, cervical smear tests, and childhood immunizations, for each member of the household, was attached to the front of the records of each patient in the deprived community.
   - As each item was completed, the date was recorded on the card.
   - The card prompted doctors to discuss any outstanding preventive care at each consultation.
   - Copies of the updated cards were supplied to the health visitors for use on home visits.

- Letters were sent to the senior female member of each household describing the practice policy on preventive care and listing the preventive record for each member of the household.
- The practice nurse reorganized her day to give immediate attention to deprived patients.
- Receptionists gave prompt attention to patients who telephoned.
- Progress was monitored every three months, and each GP was issued with a set of tables showing coverage of the various items of preventive care.
- Progress and problems were discussed regularly at practice meetings.
- Pre-arranged home visits were made jointly by doctors and health visitors to provide outstanding preventive care to those who had failed to attend the relevant clinics.

5. The results of all this activity were very encouraging:
   - childhood immunization improved;
   - cervical smear rates improved;
   - use of contraception improved;
   - anti-tetanus immunization increased;
   - blood pressure measurement increased;
   - urine analysis increased;
   - attendance at preventive health checks increased;
   - recording of smoking habits increased.

By the end of the fifteen-month programme, the deprived patients had a slightly better record for many of the preventive procedures than the endowed group.

whole range of social and economic policies and modifying or changing these policies where necessary.

For example, increasing the tax on tobacco might be considered to be the most effective way of reducing smoking and this policy might be accompanied by encouragement to the tobacco industry to diversify into healthier products. At a local level, pressure could be brought upon food retailers to stock healthier products. At the level of the practice, the incidence of childhood accidents could be monitored and action taken to reduce hazards, such as dangerous road crossings or unsafe playgrounds.

None of these ideas is new and all are being put into practice in different places. Hard-pressed members of primary health care teams may not be the most appropriate people to initiate such schemes. However, because they are in a position to know more than most about the specific health problems of their local community, they have an important role to play as advocates, ensuring that health becomes an important part of the local and national political agenda.

In order to achieve this aim, general practitioners and other members of the primary health care team will need to develop strong links with their local community. They could assist local community groups to define their health needs and to press for change. Unless concerted action is taken to assist less-advantaged members of the community to take control over their own health, the problem of socio-economic inequalities in health will persist.

Summary

- Premature mortality in the lowest socio-economic groups is twice that in the highest.
- Social class inequalities in health are widening.
- Regional differences in health are only partly explained by social class differences.
- Unemployment is a cause of ill-health.
- Smoking and abuse of alcohol are more common among those in the lowest social classes.
- Asian ethnic groups have a greater risk of heart attacks, type II diabetes and tuberculosis.
- Lifestyle explains only part of the social class differences in health.
- In tackling inequalities in health, primary care must pay attention to understanding, targeting and advocacy.
- Opportunistic screening programmes may result in 'inverse care—those most in need being least likely to receive it'.
- Inequalities in health necessitate a comprehensive public health approach, with Government, health authority, and community action complementing the efforts of primary care.

References and further reading

Cornwell, J. (1984). *Hard-earned lives: accounts of health and illness from East London.* Tavistock, London.

Coulter, A. (1987). Lifestyles and social class: implications for primary care. *Journal of the Royal College of General Practitioners*, **37**, 533–6.

Cox, B. D. *et al.* (1987). *The health and lifestyle survey.* Health Promotion Research Trust, London.

Davey Smith, G., Bartley, M., and Blane, D. (1990). The Black report on socio-economic inequalities in health 10 years on. *British Medical Journal*, **301**, 373–7.

Delamotte, T. (1991). Social class and mortality in Britain. *British Medical Journal*, **303** 1046–50.

Graham, H. (1984). *Women, health and the family.* Wheatsheaf, Brighton.

Logan, W. P. D. (1982). *Cancer mortality by occupation and social class 1851–1971*, IARC Scientific Publication No 36. HMSO, London.

Marmot, M. G. and McDowall, M. E. (1986). Mortality decline and widening social inequalities *The Lancet*, **ii**, 274–6.

Marsh, E. N. and Channing, D. M. (1988). Narrowing the gap between a deprived and an endowed community. *British Medical Journal*, **296**, 173–6.

OPCS (1986*a*). *Mortality statistics, perinatal and infant: social and biological factors for 1984.* HMSO, London.

OPCS (1986*b*). *Registrar General's decennial supplement on occupational mortality 1979–83.* HMSO, London.

Smith, A. and Jacobson, B. (1988). *The nation's health: a strategy for the 1990s.* King Edward's Hospital Fund for London, London.

Smith, R. (1987). *Unemployment and health.* Oxford University Press.

Townsend, P., Davidson, N., and Whitehead, M. (eds) (1988). *Inequalities in health: the Black Report and the health divide.* Penguin, London.

Townsend, P., Phillmore, P., and Beattie, A. (1988). *Health and deprivation: inequality and the north.* Croom Helm, London.

Waller, D., Agass, M., Mant, D., Coulter, A., Fuller, A., and Jones, L. (1990). Health checks in general practice: another example of inverse care? *British Medical Journal*, **300**, 115–18.

4 Resources for prevention and health promotion

Peter Anderson

Chapter 2 of this book has set out the challenges facing primary health care. These are essentially preventing disease and promoting healthy lifestyles (see Boxes 4.1 and 4.2). '*The health of the nation*' was published by the Department of Health as the first stage in the development of a strategy to prevent disease and promote healthy lifestyles, setting healthy targets and objectives for the nation. 'The health of the nation' recognizes the importance of primary health care as a setting to help in the prevention of disease and the promotion of a healthy lifestyle. In the Appendix of this book, the structure of the new general practitioner contract, as a means of supporting prevention and health promotion activity in primary health care, is described.

Box 4.1: Disease prevention

To add years to life and life to years by reducing the incidence and impact of disease, disability, and premature death:

- coronary heart disease;
- cerebrovascular disease;
- cancer;
- sexual health.

Box 4.2: Healthy lifestyles

To support health-enhancing behaviour and reduce health-damaging behaviour so that people can achieve their maximum health potential:

- smoking;
- alcohol;
- eating;
- physical activity;
- stress.

What should our strategic aims be?

There should be four strategic aims:

(1) disease prevention (see Box 4.1);
(2) promotion of healthy lifestyles (see Box 4.2);
(3) promotion of health skills (see Box 4.3);
(4) promotion of healthy communities (see Box 4.4).

Box 4.3: Health skills

To help individuals gain the relevant knowledge and skills needed to improve health and lead socially fulfilling lives:

- knowledge;
- attitudes;
- self-confidence;
- coping and relationships;
- self-help and mutual support.

Box 4.4: Healthy communities

To improve the quality of life by encouraging social and physical environments which promote health:

- families;
- communities;
- natural environments;
- housing and habitats.

How do we approach these aims?

The World Health Organization committed itself to the goals of 'health for all' in 1977 and with the declaration of Alma-Ata on primary health care in 1978 recognized the importance of primary health care as a means to achieving health for all.

The first international conference on health promotion in industrialized countries took place in Ottawa in 1986 and recognized the importance of health promotion as a process of enabling people to increase control over and to improve their health. Health promotion action included:

- building healthy public policy;
- creating supportive environments;
- strengthening community action;
- developing personal skills;
- reorienting health services.

The member states of the European region of the World Health Organization agreed that in order to improve health in Europe, efforts should be concentrated on the promotion of healthy lifestyles, the reduction or elimination of preventable diseases, and the provision of comprehensive health coverage for the whole population, based on primary health care, with particular attention being given to at-risk groups in society and a move away from focusing on treating disease to one of avoidance of disease. As part of the health for all by the year 2000 strategy a set of 38 targets was formulated by the European Region of the WHO. The targets can be broken down into three subsets:

1. Targets for improvements in health (reducing or eliminating preventable conditions or reducing mortality).
2. Targets for activities needed to bring about these improvements in health (policies to bring about improvements in lifestyle, e.g. reducing tobacco consumption, alcohol, and drug use, reducing environmental health risks, and improving the environment).
3. Targets designed to improve the management and organization of health services, the quality of care, and the training of health workers.

Primary health care as a setting for health promotion

The World Health Organization has considered the role of primary health care in changing lifestyles. The definition of health promotion used by the WHO Regional Office for Europe is shown below.

Health promotion is the process of enabling individuals and communities to increase control over the determinants of health and thereby improve their health.

The concept of lifestyle

In the Alma-Ata report, it was stated that health promotion is a means by which individuals and communities are empowered to increase control over the determinants of health and thereby improve their health. Those involved with health promotion are therefore concerned not only with enabling the development of lifestyles and individual competence to influence factors determining health but also with community intervention to reinforce factors supporting healthy lifestyles and to change those factors preventing or prohibiting healthy lifestyles.

From prevention to health promotion

At present primary health care providers are giving personal advice to patients about behaviour. However, important though this is, such activity is largely directed at maintaining the status quo, rather than providing a broad positive approach to health promotion which accepts the importance of the environment as a major determinant of lifestyle. Health promotion aims to influence lifestyles by a combined approach influencing not only personal health behaviour but also communities. It would seem legitimate for primary health care teams to take an interest in environmental influences on health and seek to change them, while at the same time promoting appropriate personal health behaviour by individuals and families.

Implementing the health promotion approach in primary health care

The role of primary health care providers in health promotion initiatives can be summarized under the headings used in the Ottawa Charter for Health Promotion—enabling, mediating, and advocacy (see Chapter 3). The challenge is for primary health care providers to look beyond the confines of the one-to-one consultation or even of family care, and to accept that their role is to work with others to enable the community as a whole to increase its control over the determinants of health. Primary health care teams need to deal with local issues, but they can also join with other primary health care workers to initiate and support regional and national health promotion initiatives.

Demonstration projects need to be accurately described and evaluated. Others can learn from their successes and failures. It is important therefore to have effective networking so that primary health care providers can be informed of health promotion projects going on elsewhere.

Intersectoral collaboration

One of the implications of the move from prevention to health promotion is the need for intersectoral collaboration. Collaboration may take place at a number of levels. District levels are probably the most important in terms of the organization and administration of primary health care, since these two tend to deal with policy issues and can most easily liaise with local authorities. However, collaboration also needs to take place at a local level between both non-statutory and statutory agencies.

Education of health care providers for health promotion

At present many education and training curricula for primary health care providers neglect health promotion. Continuing professional education should specifically deal with the acquisition of the appropriate skills, especially those required for collaboration with other professions and with the problems of implementing programmes.

Resources and skills are needed in the following areas:

- teamworking and intersectoral working;
- lifestyle change;
- training;
- dissemination of information;
- networking;
- research.

Teamworking and intersectoral working

A multidisciplinary team (see Box 4.5) is more likely to be able to carry out broad-based health promotion activities than individual isolated practitioners. Primary health care providers will also need to develop skills in working with groups and collaborating with other professionals.

> **Box 4.5: Members of the primary health care team**
>
> Doctors
> Practice nurses
> Administrative and managerial staff
> District nurses
> Health visitors
> Midwives
> Community psychiatric nurses
> Social workers
> Psychologists
> Dieticians
> Counsellors
> Community development workers

Primary health care team workshops should follow a problem-solving model and thereby aim to encourage the development of teamwork, organizational planning skills, and to improve understanding and communication between those working together in the general practice and primary health care setting. Participants should attend as a team. A core team usually consists of a general practitioner, practice nurse, practice receptionist, practice manager, health visitor, district nurse, but can include members of the extended team. The participants have an opportunity to learn and work together as a team to achieve a common goal. The objective for the teams is to develop a plan for prevention which reflects the needs and characteristics of the population served by each practice, taking into account the organization of the practice, its available resources, and the outlook and ambitions of the different members of the primary health care team. The evaluation of the workshops has shown that they lead to improved teamwork and communication, enhanced cooperation, coordination, and understanding between different professionals, and the development of a greater capacity for planning health promotion and prevention strategies.

Health Education Authority Primary Health Care Unit team workshops are now planned at a local level either by District Health Authorities or Family Health Service Authorities. The primary health care facilitator, GP tutor, or FHSA manager will know if primary health care team workshops are being organized at a local level. Further information can be obtained from the Health Education Authority Primary Health Care Unit.

Group working

The move to prevention and health promotion requires the learning of new skills, particularly skills in group working. At a local level many health promotion units and health promotion offices can provide skills and support in group work skills.

The Health Education Authority Primary Health Care Unit is developing access to health groups organized at a local level. Access to health uses small groups facilitated by an interested member of the primary health care team to identify the health topics in which local communities have an interest. Once specific topics are identified by the group any information required may be provided by a member of the group, the health professional, or an invited speaker. If there is a need for a service the group may decide it can provide that service itself by, for example, forming a self-help group. However, the group may decide to make the need known to established service providers in order to assist development, for example to straighten a dangerous corner in the road or to hold a well-woman's clinic. Access to health groups can be targeted at geographical areas, people within a specific age range, or with a particular interest.

Intersectoral working

Intersectoral working means working together with other agencies. This can take place at a district level or at a local level. Many regional health authorities are now developing and organizing local organizing team workshops. The local organizing team (LOT) workshop aims to establish a collaborative working relationship between members of each local organizing team which will stimulate multidisciplinary educational and training activities at district or FHSA level. This is achieved through the LOT members working together to prepare a plan for organizing and implementing workshops for primary health care teams. The members of a LOT usually consist of a primary health care facilitator, public health physician, manager of FHSA, general practitioner tutor, district health education officer and community nurse manager.

Lifestyle

A key role of primary health care is to seek to enable individuals and communities to increase control over the determinants of health and thereby improve their health. Programmes and resources are therefore needed to assist change of lifestyle at both an individual level and at a community level.

Individual level: resources

Written resources serve three functions:

1. To increase effectiveness of general-pracitce-based interventions. Several studies have shown that self-help literature enhances the effectiveness of one-to-one advice.
2. To provide a structure for nurses and doctors in giving lifestyle advice. Such a structure leads on to the ability to monitor quality of prevention and health promotion activity and assist in the audit of such activity.
3. Training resources can be used as part of training programmes, e.g. vocational training.

There are many different resources available for supporting lifestyle change and giving health education information. District Health Education Units stock health education resources and materials which are available to primary health care teams. The Health Education Authority, based in London, produces a booklet listing their resources, which are available through District Health Education Units.

The Health Education Authority Primary Health Care Unit is producing a series of resources to support lifestyle change specifically designed for primary health care to enable an increase in the effectiveness of lifestyle change. There are two components to the resources: the development of a personal health record for health checks; the development of risk management packs.

The personal health record is a patient-held record of health checks that encourages and enables patients to take responsibility for their own health through: ownership of personal health data; greater understanding of their own health processes; and the development of a partnership with health professionals in which both patient and professional would set and monitor individual targets for prevention and health promotion. The record is produced with a guideline for the health professional, a summary card for the practice to record and store information for audit and monitoring purposes, and a training video in the use of the personal health record as part of health checks. The personal health record is available to primary health care teams through FHSAs and facilitators.

The risk management packs are designed to support individual advice about lifestyle change. Each pack contains a series of self-help booklets (concerning smoking, alcohol consumption, healthy eating, physical activity, and stress) for individual patients which provide the structure for the consultation. The pack also contains a guideline for the health professional in how to use the self-help booklets. The packs are available through family health service authorities and local facilitators.

Development of protocols

For health checks and risk management there is a need to develop protocols which should include targets for preventive and health promotion activity in primary health care and guidelines about audit and quality control. As part of their application for funding for health promotion clinics practices are usually required to submit protocols to their Family Health Service Authority. In their turn, Family Health Service Authorities and their medical advisors and facilitators will be able to give advice and support on the development of protocols. Many Family Health Service Authorities will work with their local public health departments and health promotion units to obtain advice on the development of protocols. At a national level guidance about protocols and their content are available from both the Royal College of Practitioners and the Health Education Authority Primary Health Care Unit.

Promoting lifestyle change at a community level

There is a need for primary health care teams to be concerned with community intervention to enforce factors supporting healthy lifestyles and to change those factors preventing or prohibiting healthy lifestyles. This could include, for example:

- promoting access to healthy food;
- community-based programmes to reduce alcohol consumption;
- programmes to reduce smoking in public places.

There are many resources in the community, both at a statutory and non-statutory level, that can assist in this process. Many health authorities and local authority environmental health departments and district health education units may produce policies, guidelines, and strategies for supporting healthy communities.

Training

The postgraduate education allowance (PGEA) has led to the development of many training opportunities in prevention and health promotion. There are many PGEA-approved courses and distance-learning packs in the topics of prevention and health promotion. A number of practices have developed teaching programmes within practices that are eligible for PGEA approval. For further support, advice, and information postgraduate deans, general practitioner tutors, FHSA medical advisors, FHSA training advisors, and primary health care facilitators can be contacted.

Health promotion facilitators

The role of health promotion facilitators or advisors is to support primary health care teams in undertaking prevention and health promotion activities. Such facilitators usually have a nursing or health visiting background and bring with them an understanding of primary health care teams. They specialize in preventive medicine, have skills in pratice organization and management, and skills in taking measurements and giving health education. They can provide support to practices which may include advice on setting up screening programmes, managing risk, and encouraging teamwork. Facilitators are now in post throughout most of the country, employed either by Family Health Service Authorities or District Authorities or joint appointments between the two organizations. To obtain support from a facilitator contact your local Family Health Service Authority.

Audit

One of the services and support that facilitators can provide is assistance with audit, which need not only be to do with health promotion. This is now supported by the development of medical audit advisory groups (MAAG). An offer of practical help can be given to primary health care teams by trained auditors who work to a strict protocol of confidentiality. For example, a 10 per cent sample of medical records can be examined by the auditors. Audits can then be standardized to enable practices to compare with others if they wish. Identities of practices, however, are not revealed in order to maintain anonymity. Audit is particularly useful as a means of assessing progress in preventive and health promotion work (see Chapter 5).

Dissemination of information

One of the problems in a developing field is to know what is going on elsewhere. There are many ways of keeping in touch and disseminating information. At a local level facilitators and Family Health Service Authorities will know about the problems and progress that different primary health care teams have in developing programmes of prevention and health promotion. Facilitators will be able to indicate how other teams have overcome problems and be able to disseminate examples of innovative projects.

At a national level journals, newsletters, and the general practice press are a useful way of identifying developmental ideas and projects.

The Health Education Authority Primary Health Care Unit has a computerized database of health promotion activity in primary health care. The database is developing but includes information on:

- ongoing research;
- examples of good practice;
- key references in the literature.

Networking

Networking means joining with other relevant professionals to initiate and support health promotion initiatives. Statutory organizations include:

- Family Health Service Authorities;
- District Health Authorities (particularly departments of public health medicine);
- District health education units;
- Local authorities (social services departments, education departments, housing departments, environmental health departments, recreation departments).

In addition, there are many non-statutory organizations within the community that may focus on:

- different population groups, e.g. women's groups, ethnic groups, disabled groups, etc.
- different topic groups, e.g. action in areas of smoking, alcohol, eating, etc.

Many local authorities have directories of non-statutory and community organizations. In addition, facilitators from the Health Authorities and District Health Authorities would be able to identify relevant community-based non-statutory groups.

Research

The research base for health promotion in primary health care needs developing and expanding. Support for research programmes can be obtained from local university departments of primary care, district departments of public health, and in some cases Family Health Service Authorities. Some Regional Health Authorities and District Health Authorities have small grant schemes to promote research in primary health care.

Several organizations, including the Royal College of General Practitioners and the HEA Primary Health Care Unit, stock and list databases of key references in the literature and databases of ongoing research. The Association of University Teachers of General Practice is a helpful forum for disseminating research findings.

Useful addresses

Royal College of General Practitioners
14 Princes Gate
Hyde Park
London SW7 1PU

Health Education Authority National Unit for Health Promotion in Primary Health Care
Churchill Hospital
Oxford
OX3 7LS

Health Education Board for Scotland
Woodburn House
Canaan Lane
Edinburgh EH10 4SG

Health Promotion Authority for Wales
8th Floor
Brunel House
2 Fitzallen Road
Cardiff CF2 1EB

Health Promotion Authority for Northern Ireland
The Beeches
12 Hampton Manor Drive
Belfast BT7 3EN

Health Education Authority
Hamilton House
Mabledon Place
London WC1H 9TX

Further reading

World Health Organization Regional Office for Europe (1989). *The role of primary health care in changing lifestyles.* WHO, Copenhagen.

5 Information

Martin Lawrence

Where is the knowledge we have lost in information, where is the wisdom we have lost in knowledge?

Introduction

In many practices, the mail each morning can be measured in inches rather than items; pages of printout roll off practice and health authority computers. We are in danger of being driven by data, for which we subsequently have to find a justification, rather than identifying problems and using data to help solve them. Information has become the master and not the servant.

It is essential that to review our values and re-establish control—not least in the field of preventive care. The tool we can use to help is the microcomputer, whose output has been the cause of the problem. Our strategy must centre around the correct and appropriate use of medical audit.

Information for medical audit

Medical audit can be defined as the 'assessment of the quality of medical care, together with action to modify and improve it when necessary'. It is commonly considered as a cyclical process—indeed the 'repeat' characteristic of audit is essential (see Fig. 5.1).

Some of the greatest problems, both in developing the practice of preventive care and in evaluating it, have been due to neglect of this cycle. Massive emphasis as been placed on the collection and analysis of data—important enough, but disastrous if conducted in isolation. In particular such an activity may result in the valuing of a procedure just because it can be measured, without assessing whether it is a valid indicator of good care (the testing of urine at health checks is an example), or the collection of data about achieving targets, divorced from an assessment of the significance of the figures or the effect on practice organization (cervical cytology statistics would be an example here) (Health Departments of Great Britain 1989).

Indeed, once 'agreeing and developing criteria' become accepted as major elements in audit, it also becomes clear that much information is valuable which is not numerical ('Not all that counts can be counted, and not all that

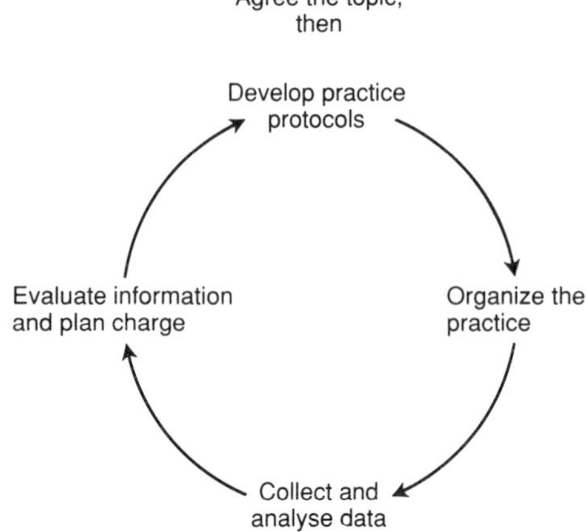

Fig. 5.1 The audit cycle.

can be counted counts'.) Thus, review of case notes, or the ascertainment of patients' views, gives information of a narrative type which may be equally important in assessing certain topics.

The value of information relating to prevention in practice can be assessed on the basis of its role in informing the audit cycle.

Develop practice protocols

In the past, the main function of medical care was reactive, and the purpose of a medical record was as an *aide-mémoire* to the doctor. In the context of preventive care this is no longer adequate. A well patient is subjected to an invasive procedure, and it is the responsibility of the doctor to ensure that this is done systematically according to a considered management plan and assessed against defined criteria;

Practice protocols for the identification of risk factors, for the management of the findings, and for the assessment of performance, need to be agreed and written. Such protocols should be kept available to all primary care team members as invaluable reference information. Only on the basis of such agreed protocols can systematic and consistent care be provided and evaluated.

The implementation of the protocol involves development of the medical record. Haphazard notes need to be replaced by a structured record which prompts the doctor or the nurse to complete the appropriate procedures, and enables the information to be recorded in a way that is repeatable, retrievable for use in patient care, and analysable in evaluation. Such a record organizes the 'information in' phase.

This organization of the record can be done by the use of a dedicated flow card (see Fig. 5.2) in the notes (Fullard *et al.* 1987). a summary grid stuck on the outside of a patient's A4 record has also been described (Marsh and Channing 1988). These are excellent for recording initial findings—they become increasingly clumsy for follow-up, and are extremely laborious to

HEALTH SUMMARY **MALE**

Name JAMES SMITH

D.O.B.	5-7-36	SMWD	M	No.	

Own Occupation	MEDICAL ILLUSTRATOR
Partner's Occupation	SECRETARIAL

Date 5-3-89	Date 12-3-89	Date 26-3-89	
1st B/P 175/105	2nd B/P 165/100	3rd B/P 170/100	Mean if applicable

Weight 12ST 4lb	Ideal Weight 11ST 10lb	Height 5'8"

Smoker	Cigarettes	Pipe	Since 19
(Non Smoker)	Never	Stopped 19	

Family History of CVA or MI	MOTHER + 63YR, CVA.

Diabetes	Yes	Insulin	OHD	Diet
	(No)			

Date of Tetanus	1st	2nd	3rd	Booster 7-7-82

Urine Date 12-3-89	Protein NIL	Sugar NIL

Alcohol	35 UNITS/WK

Allergies	/

Notes / Past Operations

12-3-89. CHOLESTEROL 7.8.
FOR F/U DIET/ALCOHOL/WEIGHT REDUCTION.

Fig. 5.2 Health summary.

use for audit because individual sets of notes have to be examined. It is almost impossible to identify omissions, i.e. items that have not been carried out.

By contrast a dedicated *computer* screen (see Fig. 5.3) can be available on any desk in a practice simultaneously, provides an everpresent prompt to encourage compliance with the protocol, can be repeatedly updated while retaining historic data, and is always for audit. The microcomputer can also contain further aids to management. For instance it can be programmed to provide the body mass index from height and weight; or it can calculate a risk score from a collection of separate risk factors. This type of processed information aids decisionmaking with regard to management or follow-up.

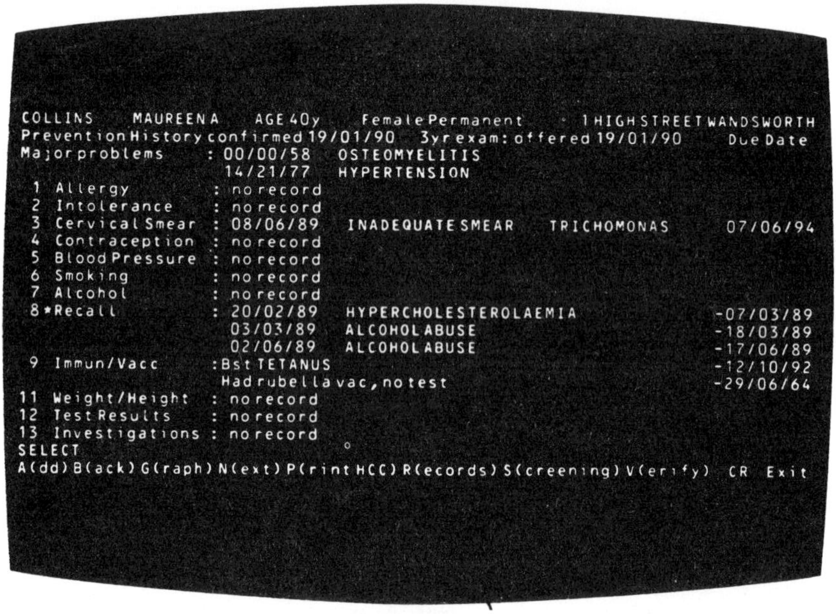

```
COLLINS    MAUREEN A    AGE 40y    Female Permanent    1 HIGH STREET WANDSWORTH
Prevention History confirmed 19/01/90   3yr exam: offered 19/01/90    Due Date
Major problems       : 00/00/58   OSTEOMYELITIS
                       14/21/77   HYPERTENSION
 1 Allergy           : no record
 2 Intolerance       : no record
 3 Cervical Smear    : 08/06/89   INADEQUATE SMEAR    TRICHOMONAS    07/06/94
 4 Contraception     : no record
 5 Blood Pressure    : no record
 6 Smoking           : no record
 7 Alcohol           : no record
 8*Recall            : 20/02/89   HYPERCHOLESTEROLAEMIA             -07/03/89
                       03/03/89   ALCOHOL ABUSE                     -18/03/89
                       02/06/89   ALCOHOL ABUSE                     -17/06/89
 9 Immun/Vacc        :Bst TETANUS                                   -12/10/92
                      Had rubella vac, no test                      -29/06/64
11 Weight/Height     : no record
12 Test Results      : no record
13 Investigations    : no record
SELECT
A(dd) B(ack) G(raph) N(ext) P(rint HCC) R(ecords) S(creening) V(erify)  CR  Exit
```

Fig. 5.3

Organize the practice

Once a preventive activity has been agreed as important, and a protocol drawn up for its management, the team must consider how best to organize the practice to deliver the care (Pritchard *et al.* 1984). Such organization depends on the item involved—immunization by call to a well-baby clinic, blood pressure measurement by opportunistic screening and referral of raised levels to an assessment clinic, cervical cytology by call/recall letter, and so on.

Such organization requires information both on the practice, in terms of time, skills, and space available; and on the patients in terms of numbers at risk, names and addresses, and the existing knowledge of each patient's risk status. Up to 10 years ago, this was largely managed on a card index basis. Practices had age–sex registers which were either sublabelled for certain procedures, or separate card indexes were set up for different items—thus, one for cervical cytology recall, one for health checks, and so on. With great application the system could be made to work and could also be audited, but the double entry was considerable, and the speed too slow. Again the microcomputer can be used to rationalize the problem. No longer are separate registers required, any register can be generated at any time by searching the practice list for the required characteristic. So for instance, a search of women aged 25–64 years gives an estimate of the workload for a wellwomen clinic; a sub-search will show how many of them are overdue for the service, or due in the next month; and a word processor can generate letters of invitation. Information for management and the process of management can be integrated.

Collection and analysis of data

Quality of care can be assessed from a combination of the criteria for assessment and the level of performance in attaining those criteria. The purpose of collecting data is to measure the level of performance in the attainment of each criterion. As such it is a major task and fraught with problems.

- The criteria have to be stated clearly, or there may be differences between observers. For instance, some may include ages 25–35 years, some 25–34 years; some may add hysterectomy to smears in calculating the proportion of total women accounted for, some may calculate the women who have had a cervical smear as a proportion of the total less those who have had hysterectomy. Such variations occur between practices or within practices over time.
- The activity must be conducted repeatedly, which is the only way to evaluate change. This can constitute a repeated demand on time.
- There is a temptation for doctors to believe that they are the only people capable of collecting and understanding data. Yet data collection only decreases their time further. Many members of the primary health care team are capable of audit data collection, and can derive great interest from and an improvement in morale by being given this responsibility and also by being included in the evaluation.
- There may be problems with sampling if the whole practice cannot be searched. The result is an approximation; and those patients known to have been missed for a procedure cannot be identified.

An early way of conducting this type of data analysis was by sampling records using a recording instrument—such as the practice activity analysis sheets produced by the RCGP research unit at Birmingham (Crombie and

Fleming 1988). These exercises provided interesting comparisons between practices but were subject to all the disadvantages listed above.

Data analysis is an area in which the microcomputer is an invaluable tool. For example, an audit of preventive procedures has been written by the author, which runs on a single command, and so takes almost no time to set up (Lawrence *et al.* 1990). The practice list is broken down for many preventive procedures such as immunization, blood pressure recording, smears, and smoking habit. The analysis is uniform across practices who can then exchange data on performance; and uniform within a practice over time, so the practice can monitor change. Moreover, the names and addresses of the patients shown to have been omitted on procedures can be identified and the services offered. This type of data analysis is very helpful for comparative and repeated analysis: it does not provide practices with the facilities to choose their topic, a desirable feature of audit. Report generators should enable that function to be carried out.

Evaluation and assessment

Evaluation and assessment are areas in which microcomputers are of no help! But it is critical to emphasize this step, because it is one often ignored. All too frequently data are analysed, put in a report, and forgotten. The essential step in making the information useful is to evaluate it and plan to develop the practice accordingly, *either* by reorganizing the practice to do better *or* by reviewing criteria (which may have been too easy to attain and need hardening up, or may not have been attained possibly because they were clinically irrelevant). This step enables the information to become a useful dynamic medium for the development of more relevant and better-quality care—it turns information into knowledge, and is even a start for turning knowledge into wisdom!

Thus information considered in relationship to audit ensures:

- that information sought is relevant and useful;
- that information is used to improve patient care;
- that failures in care are used to direct educational effort;
- that morale improves from seeing the positive use of information, rather than deteriorates from drowning in it;
- that the profession is seen to be assessing quality and therefore is accountable.

Practice reports

The ultimate in information provision in many practices is the annual practice report. This is a compilation about the practice both narrative (history, description, and educational activities) and analytic (such as consultation, visit or referral rates, preventive care, and chronic disease audits) (see

> **Box 5.1: Essentials of a practice report**
>
> Aims of the practice
> Description of the practice.
> Reports of present activity:
> • narrative;
> • numerical.
> Evaluation of achievement.
> Plans for next year.

Box 5.1). As in any good audit exercise it is essential that the report begins with the practice team's aims, and ends with objectives for the coming year (Pereira Gray 1985).

But practice takes place not in a vacuum but in the community and within the context of a wider health service. Other services and uses of information must be considered.

Information for patients

The practice report is an excellent document for presentation to the practice's patients. It may be necessary to abridge certain areas, if there have been major areas of deficiency honestly addressed, or if the report contains confidential or financial information. But publication of a report will improve relationships and satisfy accountability.

Patient access to records is an area of contention. Some practices give patients full access always, some never, some only under supervision. The microcomputer certainly facilitates patients receiving a printed subset, and this has been shown to be acceptable and to improve uptake in preventive care (Lawrence 1986). It is likely that smart cards will be available in the near future.

Clinical information for patients is available on leaflet from health education units, pharmaceutical firms, or by practices developing their own. National self-help groups provide very useful information to those with specific conditions. And directly accessible information is increasingly becoming available electronically on Meditel or Healthline for instance.

Information from health authorities

This is currently sparse, but should soon become better both in usefulness and volume. At present it is the general practitioners who are obliged to count referrals and pathology requests and deliver the information back to the health authority. Soon such information should be available in hospitals for feedback to primary care teams, who will be able to absorb it as part of their practice profiles. FHSAs already have a great deal of information about practice structure and about items generating claims. This information should come back to practices.

Information for health authorities

Information passes to health authorities on two bases: monitoring and medical audit. The two exercises are entirely different and have differing implications.

The objectives of the health authorities in carrying out external audit, or monitoring, are to demonstrate the attainment of quality of care and to assess practices for payment. The objective of practices in supplying the data will be to demonstrate achievement in order to justify payment.

The aim of medical audit is to improve care by means of education. The exercise is confidential and the objective of the practice in collecting the data is to demonstrate deficiencies that can be remedied.

1. Monitoring. Information required for the monitoring exercise is stipulated by the authority and relates to the structure or the process of a practice. Items of structure have to be supplied to obtain reimbursement—such as for rent or staff. Items of process are needed to justify payment for attaining targets or to satisfy terms of service (Health Departments of Great Britain 1989). Change will be effective because it is mediated by financial incentives, but the exercise may not be relevant to the practice, and there is no incentive for the honest addressing of deficiency.

2. Audit. Information for audit must be kept confidential, or the exercise cannot work. To achieve this, medical audit advisory groups are to be established by each FHSA; these are professional, independent committees with an obligation to preserve the confidentiality of both patients and doctors (Department of Health 1990). Practices can choose the topics that they wish to review, but any detailed information they choose to share with the MAAG will go no further: the authority must only receive 'the general results of audit'. Thus changes can be mediated only through education, but the exercise is relevant to the practice.

Information for professional development and education

The assessment of quality of care through audit is liable to reveal deficiency which necessitates education. This education will be more relevant for being driven by demonstrated need, but will generate demand for resources, for the education of general practitioners and other practice staff. Courses are increasingly available, but information is also more readily available in practice, again mediated by electronics.

- Practice libraries are certainly more comprehensive but will soon be supplemented by on-line information, via the microcomputer terminal. The Oxford System of Medicine is being produced by OUP, based on an electronic *Oxford Textbook of Medicine*, and supplemented by reference information on travel requirements, drugs, fitness to drive, terms of service, and so on.
- Searching of libraries and journals can now be conducted by Medline an electronic *Index Medicus*. This is now available on CD and can be found in most postgraduate centres and academic departments.
- Distance learning has been produced by several academic bodies. The Open University has developed courses based on videos and workbooks. The RCGP runs CASE, a system for case analysis with feedback.

Of course such in-practice facilities cannot replace the need for courses, reading, and peer discussion. But they increasingly enable practitioners to review their criteria for patient management, that basic and essential step in medical audit.

Summary

Information serves a number of functions for primary care teams. Types of information are summarized in Box 5.2.

Box 5.2: Types of information

Information for managing illness episodes:
- the medical record

Information for proactive care:
- practice protocols and audits.

Information for practice population management:
- data from FHSA and DHA sources;
- OPCS socio-economic data;
- PACT (Prescribing analysis and cost).

Information for patients:
- practice generated; practice reports;
- self-help groups.

Support information for professionals:
- printed, journals and books;
- electronic, Oxford System of Medicine and Medline;
- distance learning

Information drives the audit cycle. Information to be collected is identified when criteria are set and protocols are developed and the development of audit has an influence on both practice organization and the way in which data are collected and analysed. Focusing on audit helps primary care teams improve their information systems because the use of information for evaluation and assessment makes the information more relevant and useful and this helps to maintain and improve the quality of the information collected. Information collected for audit can also be used for practice reports.

Patients have increasing expectations about the information they should receive. Most practices now accept the need to provide clinical information for patients, to complement the advice given during the consultation. The 1990s will see developments in the debate concerning access of patients to that key source of information, the patient record.

Primary health care teams and health authorities exchange information. That from health authorities is currently sparse but improving. The information provided for health authorities is provided to allow them to monitor the work of the practice, but information for audit should remain the confidential property of the primary care team.

Finally, information should not be seen simply as a means of making primary care teams function more effectively. It could also help individuals with their own professional development and education.

References

Crombie, D. L. and Fleming, D. M. (1988). *Practice activity analysis*, Royal College of General Practitioners, occasional paper 41. RCGP, London.

Department of Health (1990). *Medical audit in the family practitioner services*, Health Circular HC(FP)(90)8. Department of Health, London.

Fullard, E. M., Fowler, G. H., and Gray, J. A. M. (1987). Promoting prevention in primary care: controlled trial of low technology, low cost approach. *British Medical Journal*, **294**, 1080–2.

Health Departments of Great Britain (1989). *General practice in the National Health Services: the 1990 contract*. HMSO, London.

Lawrence, M. S. (1986). A computer generated patient held health check card. *Journal of the Royal College of General Practitioners*, **36**, 4458–60.

Lawrence, M. S., Coulter, A., and Jones, L. (1990). A total audit of preventive procedures in 45 practices caring for 430,000 patients. *British Medical Journal*, **300**, 1501–3.

Marsh, G. N. and Channing, D. M. (1988). Narrowing the health gap between the deprived and an endowed community. *British Medical Journal*, **296**, 173–6.

Pereira Gray, D. (1985). Practice annual reports. *Medical Annual*, 285–300.

Pritchard, P. M., Low, K., and Whalen, M. (1984). *Management in general practice*. Oxford University Press.

Further reading

Westcott, R. and Jones, R. V. H. (ed.) (1988). *Information handling in general practice.* Croom Helm, London.

6 Communication

Theo Schofield

All communication has a purpose, and the purposes for which people and their doctors or nurses communicate reflect their needs and their values. In this chapter, the possible purposes of communication in prevention and health promotion, the values that underline our choice of purpose, and ways that these can be achieved effectively will be considered.

Purposes of communication

Health promotion can have three aims: the prevention of disease; the encouragement of healthy lifestyles; and the promotion of an individual's choice and control over their life and health.

Examples of communication directed towards the prevention of disease include encouraging people to take up items of preventive care, such as immunizations or cervical screening, or to adhere to the medical management of high-risk conditions, such as hypertension or diabetes. The underlying model is a medical one and the aim is to maximize compliance.

Health professionals now have a formidable list of so-called 'health' behaviours in relation to many aspects of our lives including smoking, eating, drinking, exercise, personal relationships, and even our sexual behaviour. Moreover, epidemiologists argue that to make any impact on public healthy the majority of people need to change their ways. Communication to encourage healthy lifestyles is essentially persuasive and its aim is to achieve a change in behaviour.

The third aim of health promotion is to increase people's autonomy and control over their own lives and health. This means not only that people are aware of the range of options from which they can choose and of the criteria on which to base that choice, but also that they possess the ability and power to make choices and to evaluate the consequences. The purpose of communication is therefore enablement; the aim is to increase the competence of individuals and communities.

Values and communication

There is an inherent conflict between seeking patients' compliance with medical care or encouraging the adoption of healthy lifestyles and encouraging individuals to make their own choices, which may be different to those preferred by health professionals.

This conflict revolves around two questions:

1. What does it mean to be healthy?
2. Where does power and responsibility for health lie?

Crawford (1984) has argued that there are two prevailing views of the meaning of health. The first is health as the absence of disease, which can be achieved by discipline and self-control, adopting healthy behaviours, and avoiding unhealthy ones. This view of 'working to be healthy' fits with the value that society places on individual responsibility and self-control. The second view is of health as release, i.e. being healthy is being able to do what you want to do, when you want to do it and being free of worries, particularly about health. Being involved with health care is in itself unhealthy. This view of health reflects a society dedicated to consuming the good life.

There are conflicts between these two views of health within everyone. Should health professionals seek to impose their own model of health or are they prepared not just to recognize but to accept and support different views of health? This leads to a second question: where does the power and responsibility for health lie?

The traditional model is of a knowledgeable and beneficent health profession knowing and doing what is best for other people. Owing to the power that knowledge brings, members of the health professions are able to plan preventive care services and to lay claim to a large proportion of the resources devoted to health promotion. At an individual level this power can be used to advocate compliance and lifestyle change.

The alternative view is that power and responsibility lie with individuals who make their own choices about health behaviour and the use of health services. If this view is accepted, the aim of health professionals should be to share knowledge to enable patients to make informed choices. Health professionals must be able to accept that some patients can make choices that differ from those advised and to avoid blaming patients if the consequences of their choices are not satisfactory.

A third view is that, within society, many individuals are unaccustomed and unable to control many aspects of their lifestyle. Exhortations to take individual responsibility without enabling people to have more control is ineffective at best and demoralizing at worst.

If health professionals recognize that patients are people, who may have beliefs about health very different from their own, and, if the role of a health professional is to enhance patients' autonomy and control over their own health, a patient-centred approach to communication will be adopted. Although this conclusion can be applied to all communication by health professionals, it is particularly relevant to communication between individuals, i.e. within a patient consultation, which is the subject of the rest of this chapter.

Patient-centred communication

Communication between doctors, nurses or other health professionals and their patients is always a two-way process; in much of the research in which attempts have been made to relate actions or behaviours of the professional with outcomes for the patient, the active contribution that the patient can make has been ignored. Communication is patient-centred if it maximizes the patient's involvement (see Box 6.1).

Box 6.1: The characteristics of patient-centred communication

- Patients' reasons for attending and their agenda are established and met.
- Patients' ideas about their health and health care are explored and respected.
- Explanations are given that react to and build on those ideas and enable patients to develop their own understanding.
- Reasons for choices are explained so that patients' abilities to make their own decisions and evaluate their own care are enhanced.
- The decision making is shared and patients are encouraged to take appropriate responsibility.
- Support that is offered is directed at improving patients' ability to exercise their own choices rather than to create dependence.

Reasons for adopting a patient-centred approach

There are several reasons for adopting a patient-centred approach:

1. The potential of communication to be therapeutic. Allowing patients to express their concerns and for a health professional to respond to them by giving patients information that enables them to understand their experience can reduce patients' anxiety and increase their sense of control. This is particularly important in the context of screening in which the finding of a pre-

viously undetected problem, such as high blood pressure or an abnormal cervical smear, can turn someone who considered himself to be healthy into someone who believes he has a disese with all its attendant anxieties.

2. Patients expect to be more involved in their own care and will be more satisfied if they are. In the event of a mishap, patients may be less likely to enter into litigation using the grounds that: 'If I had been warned this might happen, I would have never taken the treatment'. However, advocating the active participation of patients in decisions about their care is not the same as consumerism in which the customers' only choice is among different providers of care with no other influence on the provider.

3. When advocating the adoption of healthier lifestyles, fully informed mutual decision-making is much more likely to be effective. To make changes, patients need to know how and why as well as what to do. Non-compliance outside the consulting room may be the only option for patients who have not been involved in making the decisions within it. Attempts to influence people's behaviour must be based on an understanding of the reasons for their behaviour and why they might change.

Models of behaviour change

Several models can be used to understand why people change their behaviour.

Health education The simplest form of this approach is to work on the assumption that if people were made aware of the risks they would change their behaviour. Although evidence to the contrary abounds, this approach continues to be used in media campaigns and in spelling out risks to individual patients. Inducing fear is more likely to be counterproductive because it can lead to the denial and ignoring of problems altogether.

Health education must attain a series of goals, ranging from raising people's consciousness and providing information about problems, to making patients aware of the relevance of this information to themselves, thereby enabling them to change their attitudes and ultimately make decisions that will lead to a change in behaviour. This is a time-consuming process, both for the provider of the education and for its recipient, and may be accomplished only by repeated educational inputs.

Behavioural learning In this model it is the rewards that people receive for a particular behaviour that reinforce or perpetuate it: the more immediate the reward and the more closely related to the behaviour, the more powerful this approach is. Once a behaviour is learnt, rewards will not need to be provided on every occasion, but good behaviours will tend to be extinguished if all rewards are withdrawn. Many 'unhealthy' behaviours poduce immediate gratification, for example, a 'rich' meal. The change in weight next morning, or at next week's slimming group, or the praise of a partner may affect behaviour, but the prospect of reducing the risk of arthritis (caused by obesity) in later years will not.

Locus of control People differ in their perceptions of who or what controls their health. Those who have an internal locus of control believe that they control events, whereas someone with an external locus of control tends to be fatalistic, believing events are determined by chance, or dependent on powerful others such as health professionals. People who believe they are in control of their own health are more likely to adopt healthy behaviours.

Social factors The environment and social group within which people live have major effects on their behaviour and their ability to change it. Behaviours are learnt intitially from the family but very soon the influence of peer groups becomes important; peer-group approval is a powerful pressure to maintain certain behaviours. The social environment can provide support and opportunities for change or, particularly for the less advantaged socio-economic groups, powerful constraints militating against it. Examples not only include accessibility to sports facilities and the availability and cost of healthy foods, but also the amount of personal space, both physical and emotional, individuals have in which to make decisions about their life.

The health belief model In this model, which was first described by Becker (1974), an attempt was made to bring together elements of educational, behavioural, and social models to predict the likelihood of people taking recommended preventive health actions (see Box 6.2).

In all these models, the essential point is that, although they may lead to the

Box 6.2: Key elements in the health belief model

- Health motivation: an individual's degree of interest and concern about personal health.
- Perceived susceptibility: whether the patient believes the disease is likely to affect them.
- Perceived severity: if the disease is contracted, whether it would have serious consequences or could be treated easily.
- Benefits and costs: an individual's estimates of the benefits, weighed against the cost of taking action and the barriers involved.
- Cues to action: triggers, such as an article, a health check, or a symptom, prompting behaviour change.
- Modifying factors: these include the patients' age, sex, pesonality, and social circumstances.

development of effective ways of influencing behaviour, the crucial role of the patient's set of beliefs and the environment that control their behaviour is recognized. If health professionals fail to explore and understand these factors, attempts to influence patients' behaviour will be unsuccessful.

Tasks for effective health communication

Once the aims and values of health promotion have been made clear and the necessity for adopting a patient-centred approach has been recognized, it is possible to define the tasks that should be attempted in any interview or consultation. These fall into four areas: exploration, explanation, negotiation, and support (see Box 6.3).

Box 6.3: Tasks for effective health communication

Exploration
- Patients' reasons for attending and their expectations.
- The nature of patients' problems, health behaviours, and risk factors.
- Patients' knowledge, beliefs, and concerns about their health.
- The social and other factors that influence their health behaviour.

Explanation
- Reinforce patients' positive ideas and counter any negative ideas.
- Achieve a shared understanding.
- Enable the patient to make informed choices.

Negotiation
- Explore possibilities for, and any barriers to, change.
- Define, select, and agree appropriate goals.
- Encourage the patient to take appropriate responsibility.

Support
- Provide, and encourage the patient to identify, positive reinforcement.
- Identify and use available resources.
- Arrange appropriate follow-up.

Exploration The first task is to establish the reasons why the patient has chosen to come, the issues that he or she wishes to discuss, and the patient's expectations of the interview. These may differ from the doctor's or nurse's understanding of the problem, but it is important to establish the patient's concerns before the agenda for the interview can be negotiated. For example, a woman visiting a nurse for a health check may regard her menopausal symptoms as her major problem and welcome the opportunity of talking to another female about them, whereas the nurse will be aiming to elicit information to complete a checklist of cardiovascular risk factors. Neither will feel satisfied unless these agendas are met and time is allocated accordingly.

The exploration must include not only the nature of the patient's problems—the symptoms, risk factors, and lifestyle—but also the patient's ideas and concerns about them. From the description of the models of behaviour change already described, it should be clear that this exploration should include the following: patient's awareness and knowledge of their health problems; the factors that reward or maintain patients' behaviour; patients' sense of control over their health; patients' social circumstances and the influence that they have; and patients' beliefs about their susceptibility and vulnerability to ill-health and the benefits and costs of any behaviour change.

Explanation Having obtained this information, the explanations and information given by the health professional can build on the patient's ideas, by reinforcing positive attitudes and correct information, by supplementing incomplete information, and by countering negative ideas. Although this process may appear to be time-consuming, it has a built-in economy: it removes the need to give global explanations and allows the health professional to focus on the information that a particular patient requires. The aims of the explanations are to achieve a shared understanding about health and its problems, to allow patients to attach personal meaning to their experience, and to provide the information upon which the patient can base any decisions.

Negotiation When a shared understanding has been achieved, it is possible to enter into a negotiation about future actions for both the health professional and the patient. This will involve exploring the options offered by both parties, and consideration of the opportunities for change, the barriers to change that may have to be overcome, and the support that is available or may be required. From these options goals can be selected and agreed by both parties. These goals must be specific and achievable. It is important that patients select their own goals and are committed to their achievement. It is easy, for example, to tell an overweight smoker to stop smoking and lose two stones in weight, or to play the classic game of 'Why don't you . . .?'—'Yes, but . . .'. The antithesis to this is: 'What would you like to do, and how can I help you achieve it?'

Support The fourth task to be achieved is to offer appropriate support both in a single interview and over a period of time. Positive reinforcement is essential to maintain behaviour change, and the aim of health professionals must be to help people do this for themselves. This involves the patient identifying gains; for example, changes in weight from dieting, improved exercise tolerance from stopping smoking, or an increased sense of well-being from reductions in stress. The achievement of some goals depends on measurements, such as blood pressure and serum cholesterol; consequently, feedback on progress is an essential component of follow-up.

Communication skills

Doctors, nurses, and other health professionals have a range of individual skills that can be used to achieve these tasks. It is tempting to be prescriptive about the skills that should be used—open questions good, closed questions bad—but this is an oversimplification and does not recognize individuality. The criteria for assessing communication skills must be effectiveness at achieving the tasks in an interview and appropriateness to the individual problem and patient. The effective health pofessional will have a range of skills that can be applied flexibly in different situations and will be able to establish relationships with patients that allow the tasks to be achieved.

But, nevertheless, if we wish to improve, or to help others improve, our ability to communicate, there are some behaviours that are likely to be more effective than others; for example, open and reflective questioning and active listening to explore patients' ideas and concerns, clear, jargon-free explanations to share understanding, specific and detailed setting of goals in negotiation, and positive and empathic statements to provide support.

Our approach to learning as health professionals needs to parallel our approach with our patients. We need to be able to establish the learner's agenda, identify strengths, and make positive recommendations to help overcome weaknesses. Above all, we must share our aims, and the values that inform them.

References

Becker, M. H. (1934). The health belief model and personal health behaviour. *Health Education Monographs*, **2**, 328–35.

Crawford, L. (1984). A cultural account of health: control, release and the social body. In *Issues in the political economy of health care*, (ed. J. B. McKinlay). Tavistock, New York.

Further reading

Pendleton, D. and Hasler, T. (1983). *Doctor–patient communication*. Academic, London.

7 Management of prevention

Peter Pritchard

Introduction

Success breeds success, but how to start?

Anyone implementing a programme of prevention in their practice for the first time needs it to be a success. Otherwise, further initiatives may be resisted and the innovator discredited. Can we ensure that our plans are successful by applying management knowledge and skills in order to make plans work as intended?

Applying medical knowledge about prevention, whether to an individual or to a population at risk, involves a delicate balance between the technical requirements of innovation, and the complex human factors that determine whether people will accept a change in behaviour. Technical issues in health promotion and the prevention of illness vary with the task and the context. Many have been covered elsewhere in this book. In this chapter, the focus will concentrate on the human aspects of management in the context of preventive medicine.

Managing the technical aspects of prevention

Programmes of prevention must be technically faultless. Tests must be of adequate quality, sensitivity, specificity, and predictive value (see p. 93). They must be competently performed on the target population and the results passed to patients, acted upon, and evaluated so that health is enhanced. In order to define the target population, some sort of population list is needed, such as an age–gender register. Although a manual register may be satisfactory, a computer makes the job so much easier that its use is almost obligatory. However, the way in which a computer system is implemented and used must be well managed. The interface between people and any machine raises a number of unexpected human problems which may become a serious management issue if they are ignored.

There is no place for faulty technical management.

For a programme of prevention to be technically effective, good management at many levels is essential. For example, sphygmomanometers need to be regularly serviced and checked for accuracy, and both positive and negative test results need to be communicated in an effective, humane, and 'fail-safe' manner.

Managing the human aspects of prevention

Many programmes of health promotion and disease prevention involve changing the behaviour of the subject in order to improve health. For these programmes to be effective, a more human and less technical kind of management is appropriate, using tools such as an understanding of people's health beliefs, and empathy with their feelings. Understanding and empathy can be applied at the one-to-one level, at the population level (for example, different socio-economic or ethnic groups), or at the level of an organization such as a primary health care team operating within the community.

Managing people effectively is the key, and that includes ourselves.

Developing an empathic attitude among all staff to minority groups is more likely to be successful if the practice team can be empathic towards one another. How can this be achieved? How is success measured? Can an 'empathic' team also be an effective one?

The need to see things from the viewpoint of others is particularly important in the field of prevention, where often the doctor or nurse takes the initiative in approaching the patient. This is an entirely different relationship to that of the traditional 'demand-led' encounter, and its development requires new skills from the health professional, as well as active cooperation from patients. New ground rules need to be negotiated. Compliance cannot be taken for granted.

Plain English pays off.

Doctors tend to compose invitations to patients to attend for screening in 'medical' language that people may not easily understand. This may result in poor attendance, particularly by those whose reading skills are not good or who have a language problem. It is important to elicit help, especially when the target group is of a different social class, or cultural or ethnic group, to the writer. A professional writer might be of assistance, but it is much better to have advice from the people likely to receive the letter or handout. One practice team doubled the take-up of cervical cytology screening after the invitation was reworded by a 'patient'. The Plain English Campaign have produced a excellent booklet (Cutts and Maher 1988), and they also offer an advisory language and layout service for a modest fee.

Who has a stake in the success of the project?

Implementation of the best laid of plans can be obstructed by squabbles over professional identity, territory, or control (Huntington 1981). To avoid or overcome these obstacles, team members must appreciate that: everyone's identity is important; territory—both professional and physical—may be negotiable or sacrosanct; and that everyone needs to control their 'own' part of the organization, however small.

Everyone involved in a joint effort needs to have some sense of 'ownership' of the problem and its outcome. Within any organization, there is a need to achieve a balance between rational and irrational working methods, characterized neatly by Foy (1981) as the 'yin and yang of organizations'.

Can we get the patient's anxiety level right?

By intervening in the ways that people perceive their health, health professionals raise the anxiety level of their patients. This may either encourage patients to adopt a sick role, or provoke a denial and 'flight into health' (Suchman 1965). Raising anxiety about risk may be necessary to bring about behavioural change, but that anxiety must also be allayed if the patient is to achieve a 'healthier' state than that prior to intervention.

The results of cervical cytology and breast screening programmes are often ambiguous and as such are bound to increase patient anxiety. Good management can reduce needless anxiety to a minimum; for example, if the doctor or nurse writes personally to patients to inform them of negative results as soon as they are received, this is better management than a policy of waiting for the patient to enquire. The cost of a few stamps has to be set against the missed opportunity of the doctor or nurse being the bearer of good news. Prolonging the state of anxiety increases the patient's dependency; showing concern strengthens the health-seeking relationship.

If an individual's anxiety level is already high for other reasons (such as bereavement), to what extent is it possible to justify raising it further by disclosing new areas of uncertainty? Another concern should be for the patient's dignity. Small details of privacy, for example, the nurse locking the treatment room door before taking a cervical smear, form part of good anxiety management.

Vertical or horizontal programmes

A 'vertical' programme is free-standing, and is often applied by agencies external to the primary health care organization. Examples are the World Health Organization programmes for the eradication of smallpox (successful) and malaria (failed). These programmes are tempting to governments and funding bodies as they may produce good results in the short term. However, by working independently of the primary health care team, vertical programmes may weaken it.

An effective multi-purpose system, or a quick fix?

The alternative 'horizontal' programme relies on an effective infrastructure, such as the primary health care team, which has close links with the local community and can undertake a variety of tasks, for example, immunization, family planning, and screening. However, some vertical programmes for immunizing children in very poor countries have a better success rate than the horizontal ones generally favoured in the National Health Service. These alternative strategies represent a substantial challenge to general practice—either in the realization of the potential for health promotion and preventive medicine, or to be bypassed by an impatient government and public.

Steps in management of preventive programmes

The management cycle

When putting ideas into action, there are many ways of going about it, some of which are more likely to succeed than others.

Think first—then act—then evaluate.

The most logical mechanism, which has stood the test of time, is the 'management cycle' (in actuality a spiral—see Fig. 7.1—because the end point is not the same as the start). The starting point is to perceive that action is needed. Data are then collected and the issues diagnosed. Plans are then made and implemented. Finally outcomes are evaluated and the process begins again in the light of our fresh views of problems or need. This process has much in common with the way general practitioners operate during a consultation. The trick is to apply the method in an organizational setting, by 'treating the organization like a patient', bearing in mind that diagnosis precedes treatment. The pitfall is to implement a 'favoured' solution before the issues have been explored and plans made—'a solution in search of a problem'.

Planning

In a complex environment like primary health care, planning can be a difficult task: the future is difficult to predict, and nothing remains static. The rate of change in society is more rapid than the facility with which some are able to

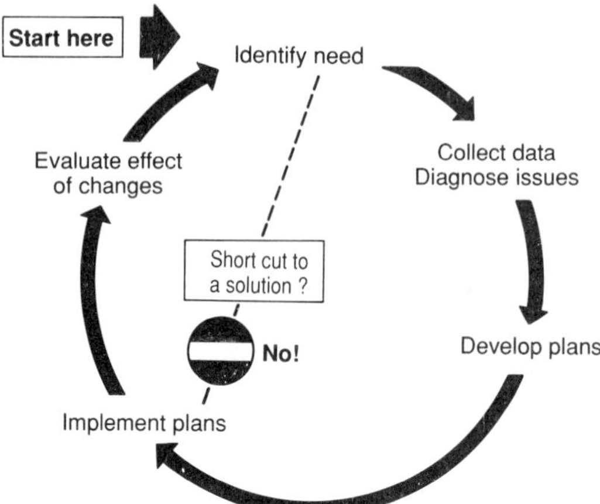

Fig. 7.1 The 'management cycle'. Management must start with the identification of need, then follow a logical cycle of actions until a review point, which initiates a further cycle. Short-circuiting the process by jumping to a solution must be resisted at all costs.

adapt. Other people may not have the same viewpoint and behave erratically. Murphy's law (if anything can go wrong it will) rules; and small disturbances in equilibrium may have disproportionately large effects, as predicted by 'catastrophe theory' (Jantsch 1980).

Build on others' success. Involve everyone affected.

Time is well spent in studying the issues, in looking at successful applications in other practices, and in making a careful appraisal of those who will be affected by the plans. All those involved must be consulted, including the patients. The most convenient source of information and cooperation is a patient participation group (Pritchard 1986, Paine 1987); those practice teams which do not have this resource, could invite an articulate patient to join the planning group as a representative. Even minimal patient representation is better than none at all. Participation at all levels is a key principle of effective management, just as it is a cornerstone of the Alma-Ata declaration (1978).

Motivating

Convincing people to cooperate with preventive measures or to change their lifestyle is a major challenge to management. Patients will not be keen to change their smoking habits if they do not believe that smoking is harmful (for example: 'My grandfather smoked like a chimney and lived to 95 in good health.'), or they regard the 'locus of control' as outside themselves (for example: 'It's all due to pollution.'). The hardest group to motivate comprises those who believe that the causes and risks of ill-health are under supernatural rather than human control.

Motivating lay staff, nurses, or medical colleagues may be equally difficult. These issues will be addressed further on p. 76.

Implementation and evaluation

Steps in implementing the plans and evaluating the outcomes need to be set out in detail. Target dates must be set by which time a planned level of implementation should have taken place. Evaluation may be easy (e.g. numbers and percentages immunized or screened) or difficult (e.g. levels of tobacco, drug, or alcohol abuse in the practice population). All, or nearly all, evaluation needs a denominator of the practice population in the form of an accurate and up-to-date age-gender register (as mentioned above).

Resources

Preventive programmes need money (capital or revenue), information, buildings, staff (numbers, knowledge, skills, attitudes, and training), and the time, enthusiasm, energy, and high morale of everyone involved.

Value for money? Why not? Money does not grow on trees.

Health services are in the process of being given more 'business orientation' in order to obtain measurable results and value for money. Trying to attach a value to one person's suffering may raise medical hackles, but the alternative approach will deny other people treatment for which they may have a more pressing need.

Primary health care has many internal resources—is it possible to tap them?

Obtaining and managing physical resources (such as buildings and money) often involves people and organizations outside general practice, and these will be considered later (p. 82). However, many of the human resources are located within the primary health care unit, the members of which are remarkably free to make their own decisions. This is another reason for concentrating on the development of human resources within the team and the locality, examples of which are described below.

Applying management to preventive medicine

Investing time in prevention

How can I? I don't have enough time as it is.

Most general practitioners say that they are short of time, and setting up the sort of preventive procedures described in this book could consume a considerable amount of time. In the long term, health promotion and preventive medicine should reduce workload, but, as is the case with money, it is important to invest now in order to make savings later.

Efficiency is doing things the right way. Effectiveness is doing the right things in the right order.

The goal should be *effective* use of time, such that time is spent wisely in order to achieve stated aims, with due concern for priorities. To achieve that ideal state the opportunity should be created in which it is possible to think out and plan the work in relation to time.

The first step might be to save some time for thinking and planning by using time *efficiently*, which means not wasting it (see Box 7.1).

Box 7.1: Ways in which time can be wasted

Putting off important tasks.	Why not do it now?
Doing too many things yourself which others could do.	Why not delegate?
Fussing over small details.	Why not forget them?
Not planning ahead.	Do we have a plan?
No clear goals/objectives.	Do we know where we are heading?
No clear priorities.	Do we have a clue?
Too many meetings.	'Groupitis' may be fun, but . . .?
Too many interruptions, e.g. visitors, telephones.	Is the stress level too high?
Too much paperwork.	Do we use short cuts?
Dealing with crises due to communication failure.	Who has to pick up the bits?
Workload unrealistically large.	Are some hard decisions needed?

Reschedule saved time quickly before it disappears.

Immediately time has been saved it must be put to good use, otherwise it will be squandered—Parkinson's law: work expands to fill the time allotted for its completion.For example, a GP might, in the first free moment, write a list of all the tasks needing to be done–today, this week, this month, this year. Each task should be classified and either *important* or *urgent*, or both. Important tasks are those relating to the main functions and goals (short and long term) of any health professional. Urgent tasks may not be important at all, but cannot wait. Once the tasks are designated as 'I' or 'U', they can be ranked in order of priority (see Box 7.2).

Box 7.2: Ranking of tasks

1. Those tasks that are important and urgent, do soon, and take enough time.
2. Those tasks that are important but not urgent, schedule time in diary or year planner—don't wait for a crisis to occur.
3. Those tasks that are urgent but not important, do soon but do them quickly.
4. Those tasks that are neither important nor urgent, question if they need doing at all or if they can be delegated.

(From Video Arts Ltd 1983.)

Try to manage time actively not just reactively.

Much of the general practitioner's traditional workload is *reactive*, in responding to demand. Preventive work involves *active* planning of time and tasks in order to achieve the aims. This shift from reactive to active ('pro-active') management is a major challenge to general practitioners and staff. Reactive management is led by demand, whereas active management seeks to achieve a goal. Unless these goals are clear and the steps toward them clearly set out, motivation will suffer, and GPs will be tempted to take the easy option of waiting for something urgent to happen.

The active manager has control of time:
the reactive manager is a slave to it.

As general practitioners, by the very nature of their work, need to be sensitive to patients' needs as expressed by demand, the shackles of reactive time cannot be thrown off too ruthlessly. The other side of the coin is that patients also have many demands on their time, which should be understood and taken into account.

Patients have time problems too; is 'time-empathy' the answer?

Empathy in the consultation, and within the organization, needs to include the dimension of time, both for the patient and the doctor.

Preventive programmes are often run within the framework of a clinic, which protects the doctor from interruption, particularly in relation to procedures; however, within a clinic, patients have to conform more closely to medical time structures that may not suit them. This may bias attendance against those who have difficulty in managing their time.

Building the team

Teams, like motor cars, do not simply come into being: they must be built.

Most preventive programmes in primary health care are team efforts. Practice nurses, in particular, take on much of the additional workload. Receptionists may need to be motivated to change their work practices, and will benefit from being regarded as full members of the primary health care team. Everyone working in the team needs to be valued for the contribution they make and for their dedication to the benefit of patients and the goals of the practice.

Every team member must be valued.
Teams need to share values and goals.

Team members, particularly those from different occupations, are likely to have different viewpoints and values. This is a source of strength, giving a broad base upon which to make decisions. However, some sharing of values and goals is essential for successful teamwork. This can be achieved only if goals and values are openly discussed, and any differences of opinion modified by negotiation. General practitioners are well placed to lead the primary health care team (in most but not all circumstances) but this leadership must be earned and not claimed as a right.

Teamwork is a mutual learning process.

Team building is a learning process which is most effective when applied to current cases with actual team members, rather than that experienced on courses remote from the workplace. Courses have a value in raising awareness, and may help team leaders or facilitators increase their skills, but may at the same time distance them from other team members. Learning together is a powerful bonding process for the whole team.

'In-house' team building works best.

Although in-house and in-team learning are the favoured options, both require time and people must be prepared to undertake it. For many it will be a threatening experience, as participants will be enabled to say all they have left unsaid, so the early team building sessions may be stormy. Help is at hand in the form of learning packages (e.g. Pritchard and Pritchard 1992).

Some team members will be competent at group work, such that outside consultant help is probably not necessary. If, however, the problems faced by the team appear formidable, an outsider with suitable skills (such as an organization development consultant) may be particularly valuable.

Team building has logical steps.

The training programme quote above focuses on task-orientated teamwork, and it is advised that questions are asked in a logical order, as shown in Box 7.3.

Box 7.3: Steps in team development

- What are our goals and tasks?
- Who does what? What are our roles, and do we need to negotiate role boundaries?
- Have we good procedures for communication and cooperation in carrying out our joint tasks?
- Are there any interpersonal problems?

Their message is that by focusing on goals, tasks, roles, and procedures a good working relationship develops, and any initial interpersonal conflicts become less important. By starting with the positive contributions that each team member can make, people begin to value each other rather than take up fixed and stereotyped opposition. If, however, the group starts by trying to sort out the interpersonal difficulties, then the actual task may never be reached! One model is the pragmatic task-oriented team: the other in the less productive therapeutic group. For further guidelines on team development see Pritchard and Pritchard (1992).

Building the organization—conceptual modelling

When the preventive or promotive project is technically complex, problems arise about the differing concepts of the medical process and how they are best tackled. For example, the people concerned with diabetes (experts, GPs, nurses, lay staff, and patients) may have different ideas about the disease process. Unless these differences are reconciled, and some common understanding reached, progress will be slow. One solution to this problem has been to use 'conceptual modelling', and this has been applied very successfully to the prevention of complications of diabetes in Sweden (Rosenqvist 1988).

Can we design our team organization to fit the job?

The starting point is to put up on a wall board all the factors affecting the problem, as seen by all the people concerned, including experts and patients. Then all these factors are linked by arrows containing a verb. For example:

good diabetic care—*requires* → careful control of blood glucose—*lessens*→ complications.

In this way a detailed picture emerges of all the factors, problems and processes as seen by all the participants. From this is built the local organization that will deliver care.

Swedish workers have found that it is more effective for each team to build its own organization, specifically to meet its own needs and problems, rather than to accept an imposed work structure. They have evaluated their work in relation to the care of diabetes and shown that locally developed plans were much more effective than centrally developed protocols applied through traditional continuing medical education. Criteria for evaluation were also developed, which have shown that care of patients is markedly improved in terms of lower rates of complications and less hospitalization.

Quality circles—a bridge between teamwork and quality assurance

The need for quality assurance is implicit in all the activities of general practice, and is referred to elsewhere in the book (Chapter 5 and p. 99). One method of improving quality of care that is finding favour is the 'quality circle'. Originally an American idea, it was applied in Japanese industry, and is now being increasingly employed in health care settings in Britain. Quality circles have much in common with the multidisciplinary team, and by focusing on quality they provide an alternative method of increasing work-effectiveness and improving teamwork that some people may prefer.

Focusing on quality will help to generate good teamwork.

Quality circles have developed useful procedures and techniques (Morland 1981) as outlined below:

Successful quality circles consist of 3–10 members from the same work unit who meet to identify and solve work-related problems in a systematic way. They usually meet for about an hour, about once a week. Each circle has a leader and a facilitator who preferably receives some training. They develop an open management style that helps to bridge any 'them' and 'us' divisions in an organization. This can have particular advantages in primary health care teams where the traditional boundaries between doctors, nurses and lay staff may inhibit working together.

The techniques that quality circles may employ include 'brainstorming', listing priorities, cause-and-effect analysis, creative thinking, choosing the best alternative, and charting results.

Management of the process of change

No-one can escape the changes occurring within our professional work and in the world outside. Anyone committed to prevention is trying to provoke change. So what steps can be taken to bring about desirable changes while minimizing the disruption that is bound to follow?

Do *we* plan our own future, or does someone else?

1. Try to build a vision of the future: for example, a future in which preventable diseases are largely controlled and the remainder effectively treated; working with an efficient happy team; earning a good income; having enough time for the family and leisure pursuits. It does not matter if these visions seem like a Utopian dream, it is important to have dreams and to share them with colleagues, and then look at ways of working towards achieving them where possible. Unless the distant goal is defined, how can we steer towards it?

Next we must tackle obstacles to successful change.

2. Identify the forces resisting change and those helping it, then concentrate on the hindering factors. What are they? How strong are they? Can they be circumvented?

The change process must be visible to all those it affects.

3. Everyone who is affected by the change must be involved and the processes of planning, implementation, and evaluation should take place at a rate that is suitable to all.

Are we capable of changing?

4. When planning change, it is important to question whether we are capable, as individuals or as an organization, to make the desired changes. If we cannot climb the steps, we are likely to fail. But once a shortfall in capability is identified, it might be remedied by engaging or retraining staff, or by taking a different route.

The checklist show in in Box 7.4 may be helpful.

Box 7.4: Checklist for managing change (from Pritchard 1984)

Diagnosis
- What is the specific need for change?
- Who could be involved or affected?
- What is the nature of the need?
- What are the possible responses/changes?

Planning
- How would we like it to be?
- What needs to change for this to happen?
- What steps are involved?
- What factors may help or hinder?

Managing
- How do we make the process visible?
- How do we manage the transition(s)?
- How do we minimize resistance?
- How do we review effectiveness:?

Delegation and training

Much preventive work in general practice depends on delegation, but poor delegation can have disastrous consequences The doctor is personally responsible for a wide range of patient care, including that carried out by employees of the practice. Will they make mistakes? Are they competent? Can we let go jobs that we enjoy doing but which do not need a doctor's skill?

Delegation is more than just telling people to do something.

The golden rules of delegation are shown in Box 7.5 (from Video Arts Ltd 1983).

Box 7.5: The golden rules of delegation

Define carefully which task to delegate, and who is to do it.
Brief or train them until they are competent and confident enough to do it.
Tell other people who may be involved that the job has been delegated, and to whom.
Be available to help if required, but do not interfere.
Allow time to check that the delegation has been effective.

Delegation must be linked to training.

Training staff is the responsibility of the practice. What cannot be arranged outside the practice must be done 'in-house'. Although it is more difficult to arrange, 'in-house' training has a number of advantages (see Box 7.6). For successful training, the teachers must be competent and be prepared to give time to assessing training needs, teaching, and evaluating the outcome (Pritchard 1988). Lunch-time teaching sessions with video or audiotapes for all interested staff are a good starting point.

Box 7.6: The advantages of 'in-house' training

It is more directly related to the needs of the job.
It involves several disciplines.
It raises confidence and morale.
It provokes discussion about the way the organization works.
It costs less.

Managing the world outside the practice

General practice is not an island.

Health promotion and preventive medicine are characterized by 'outreach' into people's lives and the communities in which they live. How can the behaviour of people and of organizations outside the practice be influenced?

Screening programmes may involve district nurses, health visitors, or any other 'attached' staff employed and managed by a different authority. How can cooperation from the managers of nurses or social workers be achieved?

'Why?' is the first question. What do we aim to achieve?

When a specific programme is being planned, the first step is to spell out the aims and proposed methods and then consult the managers concerned, to ensure that the aims are shared, the methods and targets are agreed, the resources are available, and the evaluation process confirmed.

Cooperation cannot be taken for granted. If the programme is a success, then the next cooperative venture is likely to be successful, and the practice will gain a reputation for being easy to work with.

Collaboration depends on trust which must be earned.

Working together builds mutual esteem and trust, and this improves the climate of cooperation. If we expect other people and organizations to help us in our plans, we must do the same for them. If the practice and the primary health care team respond positively to requests, a network of helpful contacts will arise—thereby creating a wider team. If doctors respond negatively, or hold on too tightly to their professional dignity and territorial exclusiveness, they will become isolated from community networks and plans will founder. Cooperation must be earned; it cannot be demanded. Five steps in managing the outside world are listed in Box 7.7.

Box 7.7: Management of the outside world

1. Understand our own and other people's organizations and viewpoints.
2. Take the initiative in communication, and build up a network of key people.
3. Build a climate of cooperation and trust by sharing common values, goals, and assumptions, thereby earning respect.
4. Ensure input from patients.
5. Avoid competitiveness, and ensure that conflict is creative not destructive.

Conclusion

First we must manage ourselves.

Management can be defined as *the application of common sense and specialized knowledge and skills to the achievement of aims now and in the future* (Pritchard *et al.* (1984). In this chapter, it has been possible to include only some fragments of specialized knowledge. Common sense can be taken for granted, but the management of others will be successful only if we can understand and manage ourselves (see Box 7.8).

> **Box 7.8: Self-management**
>
> Be clear and explicit about values and goals.
> Manage time actively and effectively.
> Be prepared to listen and act empathically.
> Involve everyone who is affected by proposals.
> Remember to evaluate both process and outcome where possible.

References and further reading

Alma-Ata declaration (1978). *Primary health care*, Report of an international conference on primary health care, Alma-Ata, USSR, 6–12 September 1978. World Health Organization–UNICEF, Geneva.

Cutts, M. and Maher, C. (1988). *The plain English story.* Plain English Campaign, Outram House, 15 Canal Street, Whaley Bridge, Stockport SK12 7LF.

Foy, N. (1981) *The yin and yang of organizations.* Grant McIntyre (Blackwells), Oxford.

Huntington, J. (1981). *Social work and general medical practice–collaboration or conflict.* Allen and Unwin, London.

Jantsch, E. (1980). *The self-organizing universe. Scientific and human implications of the emerging paradigm of evolution.* Pergamon, Oxford.

Morland, J. (1981). *Quality circles.* The Industrial Society, London.

Paine, T. (1987). How to set up a patient participation group. *British Medical Journal*, **295**, 828–9.

Pritchard, P., Low, K., and Whalen, M. (1984). *Management in general practice.*: Oxford Medical Publications.

Pritchard, P. M. M. (1986) Participation. In *Primary health care 2000*, (eds. J. Fry and J. Hasler). Churchill Livingstone, Edinburgh.

Pritchard, P. M. M. (1988). Training practice staff I and II. *Horizons: continuing education in primary care*, **2**, 217–22 (April) and 295–9 (May).

Pritchard, P. M. M. and Pritchard, J. R. (1992). *Developing teamwork in primary health care.* Oxford University Press, Oxford.

Pritchard, W. (1984). How to achieve change. In *Change: the challenge for the future*, (ed. L. Zander). Royal College of General Practitioners, London

Rosenqvist, U. (1988). Diabetes health care evaluation. In *Diabetes care as a model for primary health care*, Proceedings of WHO workshop, Karolinksa Institute, Stockholm, June 1986, (eds. R. Luft, J. Bajaj, and U. Rosenqvist). Elsevier, Amsterdam.

Rubin, I. M., Plovnick, M. S., and Fry, R. E. (1978). *Improving the coordination of care. A program for health team development.* Ballinger, Cambridge, MA.

Suchman, E. A. (1965). The stages of illness and medical care. *Journal of Health and Social Behaviour*, **5**, 114–18.

Video Arts Ltd (1983). *The unorganized manager I and II*, Film, video and booklet. Video Arts Ltd, Dumbarton House, 68 Oxford Street, London W1N 9LA. (They also publish several other training films/videos and booklets, many highly relevant in this context. For example: *If looks could kill: the power of behaviour; Meetings, bloody meetings* and *More bloody meetings; From 'No' to 'Yes': the constructive route to agreement; Managing learning 1. The concept. 2. Developing skills; All change: the management of change.*

8 Screening adults in general practice

David Mant

Introduction

Importance

General practitioners have always been involved in screening in its wider sense. Serious disease is rare in the community and all general practitioners spend their early years learning that the significance of cardinal symptoms and signs is very different outside hospital. Because disease prevalence is low, the normal diagnostic process in general practice is closely akin to screening. However, mass screening of the healthy adult population is becoming an increasingly important and time-consuming part of general practice for two reasons. First, it has been made a contractual obligation for general practitioners to perform screening tests. Second, general practitioners are having to cope with the difficulties that arise from large-scale screening programmes undertaken outside general practice—particularly from mammographic and cholesterol screening.

Only the beginning

Contractual requirements will change but screening is unlikely to go away in the foreseeable future. General practitioners have an ethical obligation to ensure that screening is done properly and that it does their patients more good than harm. Unfortunately, as with all medical interventions, screening has great capacity to do the opposite—and it will do harm unless considerable thought and care is given to evaluation, planning, and implementation. Uncritical enthusiasm is dangerous. Screening is only the beginning. The challenge is to do some sustained good to those picked up by the screen to balance against the undisputed human and resource costs involved.

Individual screening or mass education?

The risk of cardiovascular disease in the population is related to the level of plasma cholesterol. Those with the highest levels have inherited metabolic abnormalities of lipid metabolism with an associated risk of premature death up to 100 times higher than average. It seems very sensible to screen and treat these patients. However, the proponents of this *high-risk* or *individual* screening in general practice have been challenged by those who advocate a *population* strategy. The majority of cases of cardiovascular disease occur in those who are at intermediate or low risk. An individual screening strategy to identify only those at high risk has little impact on the overall cardiovascular death rate in the population as a whole.

It would be wrong to present the individual and population strategies as being mutually incompatible. A population strategy will leave a large number of individuals at very high, and perhaps unacceptable, risk of cardiovascular disease. If these individuals can be identified and successfully treated, this is an important adjunct to a population-based policy. However, in the case of cholesterol screening, the present confusion stems from indecision about whether the prime objective is to detect familial hyperlipidaemia or to give mass health education through general practice. It is also important that an individual strategy does not encourage those at relatively low risk of cardiovascular disease to believe that they are at no risk (and can indulge themselves with cream teas). In the United Kingdom even those at low relative risk are at quite high risk in global terms.

Deciding priorities

In general practice it is impossible to do everything that one would like to. There is always an endless queue of patients who would benefit from a visit because of a recent discharge from hospital, a family crisis, a recent bereavement, or a chronic disease which needs regular assessment. In practice, the most important of these visits are done while the others remain undone. Health economists have described this process in terms of 'opportunity cost'—the cost of one visit being measured in terms of the lost opportunity of doing another. Screening in general practice has a high opportunity cost. The present repayment system means that provision of adult health checks can be self-financed but the cost to the NHS remains high. Individual practices may have to forego nursing time devoted to chronic care in order to undertake screening. In order to decide priorities it is necessary to consider three major issues: the extent of the health problem which screening is trying to avert; the effectiveness of the available intervention; and the opportunity cost of providing a sustained high-quality service. The issues of effectiveness and sustainability are taken up in a later section of this chapter, but some indication of the extent of different health problems is important.

Disease importance

The screening programmes discussed in this chapter have as their primary aim the avoidance of untimely death. Figure 8.1 shows the eight most important causes of years of life lost before the age of 65 in Oxfordshire in 1989. By

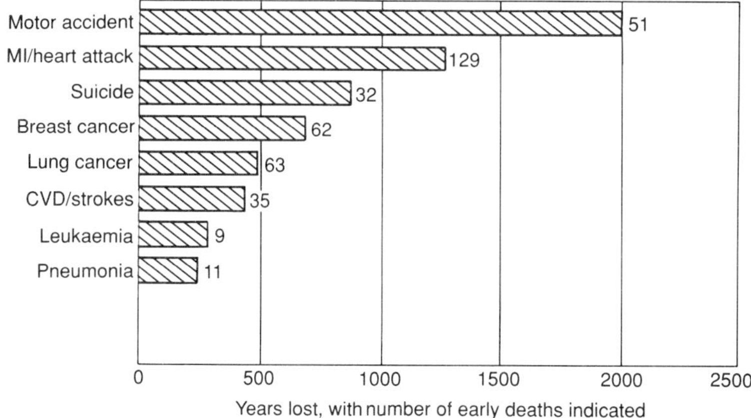

Fig. 8.1 Main causes of death and years of life lost before age 65 years in Oxfordshire in 1989. (Source: Dr R. T. Mayon-White, Consultant in Public Health Medicine, Oxfordshire Health Authority, based on mortality data supplied by the Office of Population Censuses and Surveys.)

far the most important is motor vehicle accidents. Accidents can be attributed to a number of factors, but alcohol plays a large part. The importance of cardiovascular disease and lung cancer has been known for some time. Breast cancer is also very important. Suicide remains very high on the list—accounting for more years of life lost than breast and cervical cancer together. This is an area which merits further attention, although it seems likely that there is more to be gained by ensuring that adequate follow-up is provided for those seeking help before embarking on a screening programme to identify those in need of help. Pneumonia is amenable to prevention because of the availability of an effective pneumococcal vaccine, and it has been suggested that those at risk of pneumonia by virtue of chronic lung disease or immunological deficiency should be identified by 'screening' general practice disease registers. Malignant melanoma is not in the top eight, but the incidence is increasing in the United Kingdom. It has been suggested that some form of health education which encourages people to look for early signs of malignant change in moles should be carried out in general practice (see Chapter 16).

Screening and clincal care

Although screening refers strictly to the detection of presymptomatic disease, the requirements of a high-quality clinical service dealing with chronic disease and a high-quality screening service are virtually identical.

Almost all the important questions which we should like to ask to assess whether a screening service is in the interests of a patient should also be applied to routine care in general practice.

When is screening worthwhile?

Not all screening tests are worthwhile. New screening tests are suggested, and old tests such as urinalysis recycled, on a regular basis. General practitioners must be able to decide for themselves which are worth undertaking. In 1976, a civil servant named Wilson produced a very full and detailed set of criteria. The key elements of these criteria can be grouped under three simple headings:

1. *Effectiveness.* Screening should not be undertaken unless it is known with reasonable certainty to be effective in reducing the burden of disease. If there is any doubt about the treatability of the disease at the stage diagnosed by screening (as was the case with lung cancer and breast cancer) then this can only be tested satisfactorily by a randomized controlled trial.
2. *Human costs.* The most important cost is to the patient. This can be measured both in terms of the false reassurance engendered by false negative results and the unnecessary anxiety and medical intervention occasioned by false positive results. However, there is also an opportunity cost to the practice, and it is important to assess whether the time and money spent on screening would produce a greater benefit if spent on some other aspect of clinical care.
3. *Sustainability.* This is the area in which most screening programmes fail. Resources must be available for treatment and follow-up. The quality of screening must also be sustainable. The majority of trials are done in centres of excellence with plenty of resources and well-trained individuals, and it is often difficult to achieve the same degree of quality in an every day situation over a number of years.

Assessing effectiveness

Beguiled?

Screening for pre-symptomatic disease is beguiling because at first it is extremely difficult not to do well. In the first few months or years screening programmes usually detect many new cases. The cases which are detected are invariably at an earlier and more favourable clinical stage than those presenting symptomatically. If one compares the survival rate between patients detected by screening and patients presenting clinically, the former always do much better indeed.

It is important to understand that these observations of apparent success are an inevitable part of any screening process, and they do not in any way prove that screening is in the patients' best interest. This lesson was first learned in the context of screening for lung cancer. The initial results of the Mayo lung project, which involved more than 9000 men and women, are shown in Table 8.1. This project was a randomized trial and the initial findings of the project appeared very promising, with a 25 per cent greater pick up rate for lung cancer in the intervention group and almost half the tumours being at an operable stage. The five-year survival looked even better with more than twice as many patients in the screened group than the control group still alive. However, when the cumulative nine-year lung cancer mortality rate was published it was identical in the screened and the non-screened groups. Despite the early promise, screening had been of no benefit.

Table 8.1 Results of screening for lung cancer by chest X-ray and sputum cytology. (Source: Fontana, R. S. in Miller 1985)

	Screened ($n = 4618$)	Controls ($n = 4593$)
Cases detected	167	131
Early stage	49%	31%
Five-year survival	35%	15%
Nine-year lung cancer cumulative mortality	30/1000	30/1000

Lead-time bias

How do we explain these paradoxical results? There are three explanations which play a part, to a greater or lesser extent, in any screening programme. The first explanation is that, whether or not treatment makes any difference to the natural history of the disease, patients diagnosed at screening will live longer simply because they are diagnosed before they would have presented themselves to the doctor with symptoms. In the Mayo lung project it appears that it was the advance of the date of diagnosis, rather than delay in the natural history of the disease caused by successful surgery, which was responsible for the improved five-year survival rate of the screened group. By the time the patients were diagnosed by screening it was too late for surgery to make any difference to the disease process. The technical name for the apparent improvement in survival achieved by a screening programme when treatment is ineffective and the improved survival is due only to advancement of the date of diagnosis is lead-time bias.

Length bias

There are two other reasons which explain the discrepancy between five-year survival and long-term cumulative mortality in the Mayo project. The first is the extremely worrying but common observation that screening programmes lead to an increase in incidence of the disease in question. Although this may be partly attributed to increased awareness and better reporting of the disease, some of the increase is due to the discovery of disease which would not have presented clinically during the patient's lifetime. In this sense screening programmes are creating illness.

The second associated reason is length bias. Diseases such as cancer progress at very different rates in different individuals, some illnesses apparently developing within a matter of weeks or months, while others seem to develop very slowly over many years. At any one time in any population there will be more slowly progressing than fast developing cases of disease. When one begins screening the screened population will include more patients who are likely to live longer than any group of patients from the same population who present clinically. This length bias is less intuitive but equally important as lead-time bias in misleading the enthusiast. The difficulty of estimating both biases, and the major impact they have in producing apparently favourable results in the early stages of screening, have led to the demand that no screening programme should be accepted until a positive benefit in terms of morbidity or mortality has been demonstrated in a randomized trial.

Acceptable proof

It is important to understand the need for clinical trials but also to understand that a rigorous demand for a positive randomized trial outcome cannot be absolute. Although there has been no formal trial of cervical screening, there have been a number of retrospective studies looking at the likelihood of developing cervical cancer in women who have or have not been screened. These studies show beyond reasonable doubt that screening is protective against cervical cancer and that the protective effect of screening is inversely proportional to the length of time since the last smear was done.

Even when a trial has been done, it is very difficult to demonstrate small benefits which may be of major public health importance. A good example of the difficulty of obtaining absolute proof is the UK trial of the early detection study of breast self-examination (BSE). Two of the eight centres in this study (Huddersfield and Nottingham) invited all the women in the relevant health districts to attend for teaching of BSE technique and they provided open-access clinics for the expert and rapid assessment of lumps detected. The seven-year cumulative breast cancer mortality in the two BSE areas and the four control areas was identical. However, the effect of BSE promotion was limited, with an estimated increase in the proportion of women practising BSE of only 15 per cent. At the end of the trial, the majority of women in all centres were still not practising BSE and despite the massive scale of the trial a small (up to 14 per cent) benefit could not be ruled out.

Specific programmes

Randomized control trials have been carried out to assess the effectiveness of general practice advice on stopping smoking and reducing heavy drinking. These trials have been more fully described in Chapters 9 and 11 respectively. The most important point to make here is that advice from a general practitioner backed up by supportive literature and the offer of a further appointment to discuss the success or failure is effective. Unfortunately, it is not known whether advice from a nurse is equally effective (the available evidence suggests that it is not) and the most appropriate role for the nurse might be in providing longer-term support for patients who have stopped drinking and smoking in order to achieve the sort of success rates reported from other countries such as Australia.

There is direct evidence that drug treatment of men with marked hyperlipidaemia reduces their mortality from cardiovascular disease. There is continuing debate about whether this undoubted success is offset by an increase in other causes of death consequent upon treatment with lipid-lowering drugs. This issue will not be resolved until the trials of the latest generation of drugs (statins) are completed. A recent overview of the hypertension trials confirms that treatment reduces mortality from cardiovasular disease as well as stroke.

There is now very good evidence that screening for cervical cancer and breast cancer is effective in reducing long-term mortality, but this is not true for screening for colon cancer. At the present time there are five randomized control trials of faecal occult blood testing being conducted (three in the United States, one in Scandinavia and one in Nottingham, UK) and the results of at least two of the trials are likely to be published in the near future.

The objective of routine urinalysis is unclear. The evidence suggests that it is of little benefit and has a high cost in terms of false positive results. A retrospective study of dipstick testing on 10050 healthy males receiving BUPA health checks showed a prevalence of occult haematuria of 3 per cent but very few proved to have bladder cancer or other serious abnormality. In the detection of lung and bladder cancer, cytology of sputum and urine is still in an experimental stage. Urine cytology seems to produce too many false positives without achieving a high detection rate (about 1 in 5000 screened), while doubt remains that sputum cytology detects lung cancer at a curable stage.

Ultrasound screening for ovarian cancer looks promising, but again is still at an experimental stage and takes place generally outside general practice. Screening for aortic aneurism by ultrasound is also an interesting development but is unlikely to be cost-effective unless a selective policy can be implemented. Screening for stomach cancer with double-contrast barium meal may be appropriate in other parts of the world with a very high incidence of the disease (i.e. Japan and parts of southern Europe) but is not thought to be useful in Britain and has not been subject to randomized controlled trial. Screening for testicular cancer by palpation has yet to be formally assessed, but may be important for men with a history of cryptorchidism. Screening for haemochromatosis has also been suggested recently for men and women over 30 years, with a suggested pick-up rate of 3–10/1000 screened.

Assessing costs

Human costs: four-box analysis

The major personal cost of screening is probably the anxiety and unnecessary medical investigation engendered by false positive results. It is inevitable that all screening tests will produce some false positives, and the extent of the problem can be quantified by a reconstruction of the type of four-box analysis shown in Fig. 8.2. This four-box is constructed using the predicted outcome of mammographic screening. Screening in the United Kingdom is to be based on a single lateral view of each breast and approximately eight per cent of women have some abnormality on this first X-ray which merits further investigation. These women will have further mammograms and only 1 per cent of those initially screened should need to undergo biopsy. Of women who are biopsied, about one in two will be diagnosed as suffering from breast cancer. With the additional information that for every five cases of breast cancer detected, one woman with a negative mammogram will probably present with breast cancer within the subsequent 12 months, the four-box table can be constructed.

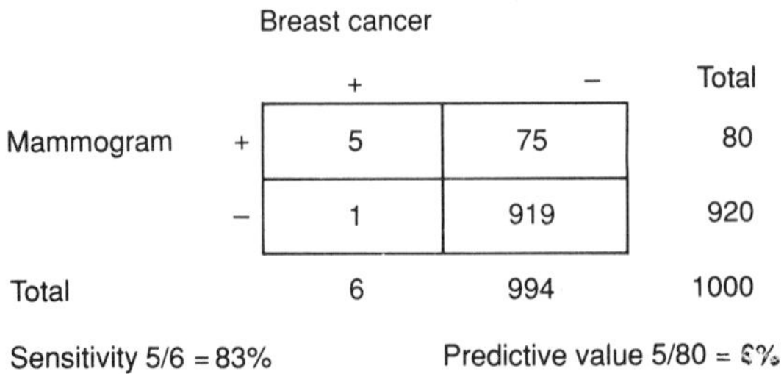

		Breast cancer +	Breast cancer –	Total
Mammogram	+	5	75	80
	–	1	919	920
Total		6	994	1000

Sensitivity 5/6 = 83% Predictive value 5/80 = 6%

Fig. 8.2 Four-box analysis: predicted result of initial mammography in 1000 women aged 50–64 years.

Sensitivity and specificity

From the figure the sensitivity (the extent to which the test successfully picks up women with cancer) and the specificity (the extent to which the test successfully confirms that women don't have cancer) can be estimated. The importance of the sensitivity is that it determines the number of false negative tests and therefore the number of women who are falsely reassured that they do not have disease. This is important because such women may delay presenting important clinical symptoms to their doctor. The specificity determines the number of false positive tests, with the attendant problems of unnecessary anxiety and investigation outlined above.

Predictive value

The most important outcome of the four-box analysis from the patient's perspective is the predictive value which in this case shows the likelihood of a woman who has a positive mammogram actually having breast cancer. The fact that, in this example, 94 out of 100 women are unnecessarily worried and further investigated would be a cause for concern.

It is of course possible to construct a four-box table for any screening or diagnostic test. It is important to understand that while the sensitivity and specificity of the test does not depend on the prevalence of disease, the clinically important predictive value does. This is because the predictive value depends on the ratio of false positive to true positive test results and the number of false positive results depends on the number of individuals screened who are healthy. This emphasizes that there is much to be gained by selectively screening a high-risk population. It also demonstrates that any diagnostic test, whether related to screening or not, will give more information about the presence of disease in a hospital than in a general practice setting simply because there are more healthy people outside than inside hospitals.

ROC curves

It is intuitively obvious that there must be some trade-off between the proportion of false positives and of false negatives produced by any screening test. If you do not wish to miss anybody with disease, you simply call every patient 'positive', thereby eliminating the false negatives at the cost of a very high number of false positives. Conversely, if you do not wish to cause any unnecessary anxiety you call everybody 'negative'. The actual relationship between the number of false positives and false negatives thrown up by any test can be characterized by what is popularly known as a 'ROC' (receiver operator characteristic) curve because it was initially devised in the training of radar operators in World War II. The point made to the radar operators was that the exact proportion of false positives and false negatives was determined by them, and that there was no 'right' or 'wrong' answer. The same principle applies to most medical screening tests. The proportion of false positives and false negatives will depend upon the training, morale, tiredness, conditions of work, and above all quality control under which the screeners work.

Minimizing human cost

A checklist of the action which must be taken to ensure that a screening test has minimized the personal cost is shown below (Box 8.1) The three key indicators are sensitivity (the extent to which the test gives false reassurance), predictive value (the extent to which the test causes unnecessary alarm), and re-attendance rate. It is also important to audit delays in the screening process as delay is an important cause of distress and must be minimized. Finally, because patients will put up with things which they feel will do them good (or which the doctor orders) even when suffering discomfort, an important role of every general practitioner is asking the patient about their experience. General practice based surveys have been important in assessing the distress caused by colorectal cancer screening and the pain and discomfort suffered by women undergoing mammography. The individual practitioner has an equally important role in assessing patient satisfaction and feeding back individual problems to those undertaking screening—be it the practice nurse or hospital consultant.

Box 8.1: Human cost indicators

Re-attendance rate
- easiest measure of consumer acceptance.

Predictive value
- indicates extent of unnecessary anxiety and intervention (the lower the value the greater the anxiety)

Sensitivity
- measures false reassurance and missed cases (the lower the value the greater the false reassurance)

Delay
- delays in the screening progress maximize distress.

Sustaining a screening programme

Advanced planning

All the screening programmes suggested have considerable opportunity costs for general practice teams. The major burden is not the screening itself but the work engendered by it, and this must be assessed before beginning to screen.

The workload incurred by offering cardiovascular health checks to patients aged 36–64 years is shown in Table 8.2.

Table 8.2 Proportion of patients aged 35–64 years requiring counselling (on smoking or diet) or clinical follow-up (for hypertension or hyperlipidaemia) as a result of health checks in general practice. (Source: ICRF OXCHECK Study Group 1991)

No specific counselling or follow-up	27%
Counselling or follow-up on one issue only	38%
Counselling or follow-up on more than one issue	35%

The implications of the cervical cancer screening programme are already well known to practices, and local experience has been that screening begets more screening. Increased emphasis on quality control in the laboratories means more requests for repeat smears because of inadequately taken or fixed smears. Increased prevalence of minor abnormalities, and particularly anxiety about the significance of papilloma virus, also means that the proportion of women being actively followed up for abnormal smears is gradually increasing.

The implications of breast cancer screening are less than initially expected, although with 8 per cent of women being recalled after the first screen general practitioners are inevitably involved in providing sympathy, support, explanation, and counselling.

The resource implications of colorectal screening by faecal occult blood testing depend upon the exact test used. With Haemoccult II the expected positivity rate is in the order of 2–4 per cent, and all these patients require counselling, further six-day haemoccult tests with diet restriction, and if these are positive, referral for colonoscopy.

Modifying workload: selective screening

If there are doubts about the ability of a practice to cope with a screening programme, it makes considerable sense to concentrate on a selected group of patients at higher risk of disease. Age and gender are easily identifiable, and invariably strong, indicators of disease risk and are useful selective criteria for all the screening tests discussed. However, it is theoretically possible to vary the screening interval according to an assessment of risk of the disease made at the first screening contact. For example, in Edinburgh, frequency of mammography was determined by asking all women attending at the first occasion about four basic risk factors. However, although this seems a very sensible and attractive idea, the predicted benefit in terms of reduced mortality is moderate and in view of the potential difficulty of organizing and explaining such a policy, it has not gained widespread acceptance.

Selective screening is already carried out for cervical cancer. Women with evidence of infection with herpes and papilloma viruses identified at screening are often invited more frequently for repeat smears than other women. (This suggestion requires careful examination because although viral infection undoubtedly indicates a higher risk of premalignancy it does not necessarily indicate a likelihood of a fast growing tumour.) Other risk factors for cervical cancer have been used only to determine the age when screening should begin (within two years of the commencement of sexual activity) and end (at age 65 years if previous smears normal and not in high-risk categories).

Selective criteria for deciding to whom to offer cholesterol screening have also been suggested. If the objective is solely to detect familial hyperlipidaemia, screening only those with a family history of premature heart disease seems sensible but Fig. 8.3 shows that no selective criteria are very much better than chance if the objective is to identify all patients with a total cholesterol greater than or equal to 8 mmol/l.

Modifying workload: repeat testing

There has been much debate about the appropriate interval between screening tests. Recommendations for cancer screening are based on an assessment of the natural history of the disease (then length of the preclinical phase during which the disease is detectable easily curable), the cost of screening, and public acceptability. Suggested intervals for cardiovascular screening have little empirical basis, and can reasonably be varied in the light of the workload which can be managed effectively in practice. In the case of cholesterol screening, a case can be made for a single measurement in early adult life.

Modify workload: follow-up protocols

The key element in determining workload is the follow-up protocol adopted. Although the practitioner has little control over follow-up of women identified as at risk by cervical screening and mammography, there is great

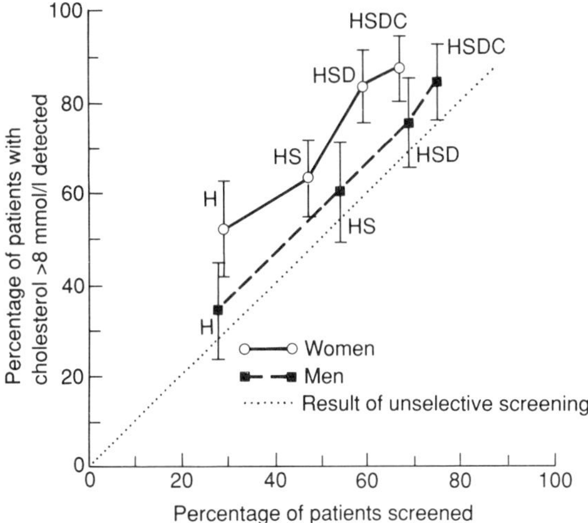

Fig. 8.3 Percentage of patients eligible for screening and percentage of patients with a total cholesterol ⩾8 mmol/l that would be detected using different criteria for screening. H = family or personal history, S = smoker, D = high-fat diet, C = clinical factors, i.e. BMI ⩾ 30 or DPB ⩾ 90. Vertical lines indicate 95 per cent confidence intervals. (Source: ICRF OXCHECK Study Group 1991)

scope for deciding on individual protocols for cardiovascular risk factors. In particular, prolonged follow-up of patients with obesity and moderate hyperlipidaemia may be both time-consuming and unproductive. A rather modest intent to follow up effectively those at highest risk may be preferable to pursuit of the unachievable.

Maintaining follow-up

In 1984 a survey of the follow-up of patients with positive smears carried out in Nottingham showed that only 19 per cent of women had satisfactory follow-up. Similar surveys of follow-up of cardiovascular risk factors, including hypertension, show a failure to adequately follow up and treat those identified as at risk. Screening without meticulous follow-up obviously does more harm than good. This requires advance planning, explicit protocols and regularly audited follow-up records. Patients must not be allowed to 'fall through the net'.

Maintaining participation

Individuals can only accept screening when offered, and the very poor population coverage in the older age groups in the UK cervical screening programme is due to the fact that women have not been offered the test rather than that they have declined to participate. However, participation rates amongst those offered screening vary between different tests and between different practices. When non-participants in a screening service are asked why they do not join in, three reasons stand out—inconvenience, dislike of the test, and fear of the outcome (Box 8.2).

Box 8.2: Reasons given for non-participation in screening tests

Inconvenience

- most non-attenders would come if minimal effort involved.

Nature of test

- pleasant, competent staff help.
- any pain or discomfort involved should be explained in advance.

Fear of outcome

- should be recognized and can be dealt with in most cases.

1. *Inconvenience.* The commonest reason given for nonparticipation with screening is 'couldn't be bothered' or 'didn't get round to it'. Such individuals can be recruited by opportunistic screening. Acceptance of bowel cancer screening is much higher following a personal approach by a general practitioner (over 60 per cent) than when the invitation is sent by post (25–50 per cent). In the context of mammographic screening for breast cancer, a trial in Aylesbury has also shown that the provision of a convenient service can reduce the 'didn't get round to it' rate. By inviting women to attend a mobile screening unit located in the practice area, very high acceptance rates approaching 90 per cent were achieved. In addition, the Aylesbury trial showed that sending a woman an invitation for screening stating a specific time for her appointment was associated with a better compliance rate than sending an invitation asking the woman to contact the surgery to make an appointment.

2. *Dislike of the test.* Another common reason given for nonparticipation is the nature of the test. It is important to try to make the experience of the test as pleasant and non-distressing as possible, particularly if rescreening is intended. However, in the context of faecal occult blood screening it is interesting to note that acceptance is no lower for Haemoccult tests (which involve fishing around in the toilet bowl) than for 'magic toilet paper' tests (which employ impregnated paper which changes colour in contact with blood). This suggests that dislike of screening does not stop patients participating if they feel it is in their own interest.

3. *Fear of outcome.* Dislike of the mechanism of the screening test is probably less important than the third common reason expressed for non-participation—fear of the outcome. It is very important to try to allay this fear by emphasizing that screening tests are designed to detect disease at a very early and curable state—in the case of cervical screening, at a premalignant phase.

Ensuring effective intervention

The key to ensuring effective intervention is staff training and support. It is not easy to take a good cervical smear or to give effective dietary or smoking cessation advice. Untrained staff (including doctors) give an ineffective service. Many FHSAs have set up training programmes, particularly for practice staff, and attendance at such a programme is likely to become a condition for payment for preventive services in the future.

Sustaining quality

This issue is of relevance to all screening programmes In cervical cancer much depends upon the assessment of a single smear: practice staff play a key role in maintaining quality, and this should be audited routinely. An equally difficult screening task which takes place in the general practice surgery is the measurement of blood pressure. The one year predictive value for an adverse cardiovascular event is about 30 per cent at diastolic blood pressure of 120 and 0.1 per cent at diastolic blood pressure of 105—i.e. it is very wide over a relatively narrow band of measurement. In this circumstance, it is vital that blood pressure is taken diligently in general practice, with proper regard for the checking of equipment, the use of the correct cuff, the rate of deflation, and the need to compare the validity of measurements between observers. Standards of treatment and follow-up should also be of high quality. Recent observations of the differences between the routine clinical measurement of blood pressure and the mean ambulatory blood pressure over a 24-hour period suggest that the former is a very crude instrument for establishing risk, and perhaps one which is overdue for improvement. However, it will be some time before the significance of these more sophisticated methods of recording will be established in terms of prognosis and until that time, sensible quality-control precautions on routine measurement should be introduced.

A good example in which a quality-assurance system has been introduced successfully in general practice is shown in Fig. 8.4. A number of practices have been undertaking measurement of cholesterol by a dry chemistry technique (in most cases using a Reflotron machine). It is widely known that such systems are extremely prone to operator error. In order to overcome this problem the Wolfson Research Laboratories in Birmingham have been operating an external quality assessment scheme for general practices and

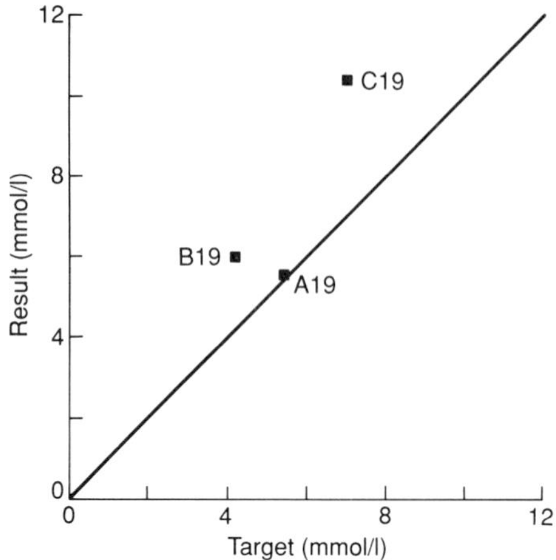

Fig. 8.4 Quality assessment in practice: example of feedback to practice on the quality of cholesterol measurement by Reflotron (see text for further details). The result and target result for each specimen are respectively for A19: 5.6 and 5.4, for B19: 6.0 and 4.2, and for C19: 10.4 and 7.0 mmol/l. The comments from the external quality assessors would run as follows:

> Your results for specimens B19 and C19 were more than 15 per cent from the target value. This suggests poor technique or carelessness and you should check the technique used against the instrument manual recommendations.
>
> We would also recommend that you contact the instrument suppliers for further advice and assistance as your results suggest a consistent problem with technique or conceivably an instrument problem.

other non-laboratory sites where cholesterol is measured. On a regular basis each participating practice is sent three human serum samples with target values linked to laboratory analyses. The general practice is asked to measure the cholesterol for each sample and to return the results to the central laboratory. The variation between the general practice and target values, with comments where appropriate, is plotted so that significant variations from the 'true' value can be detected and traced. The absolute need for such a quality assurance system (which must be supported by a programme of day-to-day quality control) is demonstrated by the range of results of 2.59–11.8 mmol/l for sample C19 reported by participating practices, compared with a target value of 6.98 mmol/l.

Summary: practical implementation

Common problems

There are a number of common practical problems which must be overcome by any general practice in the implementation of a screening programme (Box 8.3).

> **Box 8.3: Common problems in implementation**
>
> Recruitment
> - must be systematic (whether elective or opportunistic).
>
> Quality assurance
> - training of staff is the key.
>
> Time management
> - modify workload by adjusting protocols for selection and management.

1. *Recruitment.* The key to recruitment is accurate registration. Little can be done about patient mobility but practice staff can make a great contribution to maintenance of correct addresses. Practice records are likely to be more accurate than FHSA records. Telephone numbers (work and home) on the computer record are invaluable.

2. *Quality assurance.* Quality assurance depends primarily on training. However, it is important to audit the maintenance of quality in intervention and follow-up, not only for the patient's benefit but also for that of the practice staff. Everyone likes to know that they are doing a good job. Achieving this objective depends not only on good training and record keeping but also on a clear and well defined management plan for patients identified by the screening process. Quality assurance will only happen if it is planned in advance and adequate provision of time and resources are made.

3. *Time management.* There is increasing evidence that effective management of screen-detected disease such as obesity requires a magnitude of time commitment which is inconceivable within present working patterns. More research work is needed to assess the minimum resources needed for effective intervention and follow-up and a strategic decision must be made on how (and if) this work can be accommodated. This may mean deciding only to screen high-risk individuals (targeting) or redefining the roles of all members of the practice team (e.g. more reliance on nurse practitioners in both acute and preventive services). It is harder to stop screening than to start.

Implementation checklist

Before starting to screen, it is essential that the following tasks are completed (Box 8.4):

> **Box 8.4: Implementation checklist**
>
> Before screening anyone, each practice must have a:
> - screening register
> - training schedule
> - quality-control schedule
> - screening protocol
> - disease management protocol
> - audit schedule

1. *Screening register.* A screening register is mandatory. Although screening can be based on a manual age–sex register, life is made much easier with a computer. Ideally this means a computer with a terminal on every desk (including the reception desk). Computerized records make it much easier to control workload and to audit intervention and follow-up. However, a computer is only as good as its user and responsibility for updating address and screening records must be clearly identified. The need for training and professional development of reception and other practice staff cannot be overemphasized.

2. *Management protocols and training schedules.* Disease management plans (or protocols) and training schedules need to be drawn up for each disease entity to be detected by screening. Guidance and help on further reading can be found in other chapters dealing with speciic diseases.

3. *Audit and quality-control schedules.* Audit and quality control must also be planned ahead. The indicators, criteria, and performance standards to be used in audit and the frequency at which it will be done should be decided in advance. Quality control must also be scheduled: for hypertension, this means deciding how often to review sphygmomanometer function, availability of a range of cuff sizes, and blood-pressure-taking techniques; for cervical cytology it means regular review of the quality score of each individual taking smears; for those undertaking dry chemistry in the surgery (e.g. measurement of blood cholesterol or glucose) a formal quality-control protocol carried out daily is mandatory and joining a quality-control circle (such as that operated for Reflotron cholesterol measurement by the Wolfson laboratory in Birmingham) is strongly recommended.

Organization

Various organizational options can be considered (see Box 8.5) which are discussed below.

Box 8.5: Organizational decisions

- Recruitment methods
- Invitation procedures
- Clinic or surgery based screening?
- Staff roles?
- Value of targeting specific groups?

1. *Recruitment.* All screening should be systematic. Case finding and opportunism are methods of recruitment which can augment but not replace a systematic elective approach. The cost of systematic screening can be minimized if the patients are identified when consulting for some other reason, and opportunistic screening can recruit patients who would not normally respond to a telephone or letter invitation, but some systematic safety net is necessary to ensure that all patients are offered the opportunity to be screened.

2. *Invitation.* The nature of the invitation is important. This must be 'consumer oriented': clear, informative, personalized, and signed by the doctor. When inviting patients by post it must be decided whether or not to offer a fixed appointment .It has been demonstrated in two practices that a fixed appointment method is preferable to an open invitation for mobile mammographic screening, with little wastage of appointments (patients who could not keep their appointment were asked to phone for a different one). However, this needs further assessment in other practices with different geographical and social class structures.

3. *Clinics.* It is unclear whether dedicated clinics are better than integration of preventive work into routine care. Good results have certainly been reported by practitioners running asthma, diabetic, and hypertension clinics. The organization of clinics may be an important stimulus to the organization of good care of chronic disease and may also facilitate patients in achieving mutual support from fellow sufferers. On the other hand, in small practices clinics may be difficult to organize, and in all practices the case-finding element of opportunistic screening may be lost. It is obviously the quality rather than the context of care which is important and much will depend on

the reimbursement system adopted by FHSAs. At the present time much depends on local discretion.

4. *Staff roles.* Screening appears to be better when the screening task is shared between different members of the primary health care team. Practice nurses have been shown to conduct health checks more systematically than when they are left to doctors in ordinary consultations. But it is important that doctors do not 'opt out' of prevention, not only because endorsement of the nurse's activities is vital, but also because they need to be involved in the follow-up and management of those found positive on screening. The evidence for the effectiveness of intervention is also stronger for doctors.

5. *Targeting.* Targeting means selective deployment of resources. This has two advantages. First, less-privileged and high-risk patients often fail to participate in screening unless resources are specifically focused towards them. Various strategies have been suggested including the provision of additional medical and nursing time during routine consultations, and programmes to identify and approach high-risk families at their homes. Second, the cost-effectiveness and overall success of the screening programme can be improved by concentrating on the possible rather than the ideal but impractical.

Conclusion

Prevention is better than cure and screening in general practice can play an important role in reducing premature death in the UK. But enthusiasm is not enough. General practitioners often underestimate the resources needed to sustain intervention and follow-up. Detecting disease without doing anything about it is unethical. The new contract offers a challenge. Resources have been provided for manpower, training, and information technology to facilitate screening. General practitioners must provide for themselves explicit objectives and protocols. To make screening work they must audit routinely the extent to which these objectives are met and protocols observed. The most important task is not to implement new screening programmes but to make existing ones—particularly screening for breast cancer, cervix cancer, hyptertension, and smoking habit—effective.

Further reading

Goldbloom, R. and Lawrence, S. (eds.) (1990). *Preventing disease: beyond the rhetoric*. Springer, New York.

Miller, A. B. (ed.) (1985). *Screening for cancer.* Academic, New York.

Gray, J. A. M. and Vessey, M. P. (1991). *Breast cancer screening 1991: evidence and experience since the Forrest Report*, NHS Breast Screening Programme Publication. Trent RHA, Sheffield.

ICRF OXCHECK Study Group (1991). Prevalence of risk factors for heart disease in the OXCHECK study: implications for screening in general practice. *British Medical Journal*, **302**, 1057–60.

Mant, D. and Fowler, G. (1990). Urinalysis for glucose and protein: are the requirements of the new contract sensible? *British Medical Journal*, **300**, 1053–5.

Marsh, G. and Channing, D. (1988) Narrowing the gap between a deprived and an endowed community. *British Medical Journal*, **296**, 173–6.

9 Smoking
Godfrey Fowler

Smoking prevalence and changes

Since its introduction to Britain in the sixteenth century, tobacco was mainly smoked in pipes, chewed, or used as snuff until the nineteenth century. Its popularity then increased rapidly with improved methods of curing and the manufacture of cigarettes.

Changes with time

During this century tobacco consumption in the UK rose steeply until the 1970s but has since declined (Fig. 9.1). Average cigarette consumption per male in the population peaked at about ten cigarettes daily in 1945 (when about three-quarters of men smoked). For women this peak occurred in about 1975 at about six cigarettes daily (when about half of women smoked). Now about a third of both men and women smoke cigarettes and tobacco consumption is declining steeply (Fig. 9.2). But smoking is still increasing in many countries, especially in the Third World.

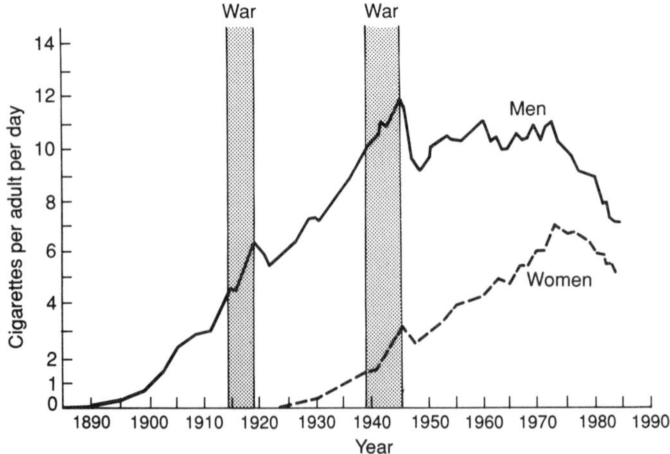

Fig. 9.1 Tobacco consumption in the UK, 1890 to 1981, given as average number of cigarettes per adult per day for men and women separately, irrespective of whether they smoke or not. (From Royal College of Physicians 1983)

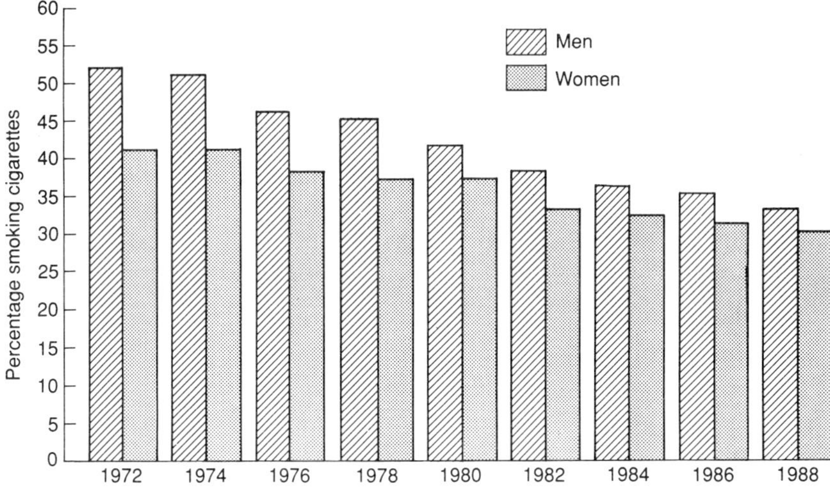

Fig. 9.2 Cigarette smoking: prevalence by sex, 1972–1988. (From OPCS 1990)

In young people smoking prevalence is not declining and in young women it seems to be increasing. The decline in smoking in women generally has been less steep than that in men.

Social class differences in smoking habit are substantial. Until about 1960, smoking was common in all socio-economic groups. Now only about one in six of professional men and women smoke compared with about half of men and a third of women in the lowest socio-economic group (Fig. 9.3).

Since the 1950s there have been major changes in cigarettes themselves as well as the more recent declines in consumption of tobacco and prevalence of smoking. Virtually all cigarettes smoked now are filter cigarettes and the average tar content today is only about half that of 30 years ago. Nicotine content is also lower.

The smoking habit

Smoking habit is almost invariably taken up in childhood and parents, siblings, and the peer group play an important part in establishing behaviour patterns.

Having a parent who smokes increases the likelihood of smoking. This has important implications for parents; those who smoke must share responsibility for their children becoming smokers. Both parents being smokers increases this influence yet further, as does having an elder brother or sister who smokes. But the greatest influence comes from friends of a similar age.

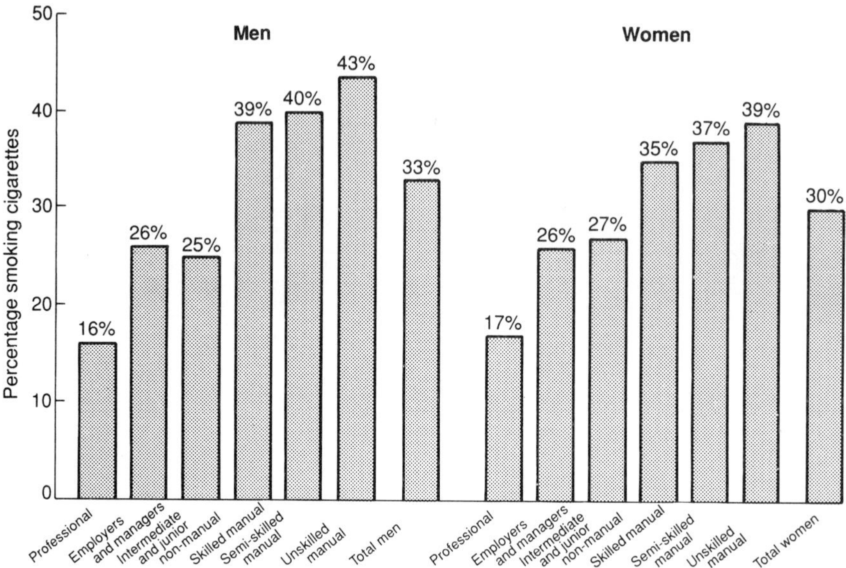

Fig. 9.3 Cigarette smoking: pevalence by sex and socio-economic group, 1988. (From OPCS 1990)

About a quarter of secondary-school children smoke, half of them regularly and about one-third of regular smokers started before the age of nine years.

Nicotine

The first experience of smoking is usually unpleasant. Owing to social influences, the habit may be confirmed, and tolerance allows the unpleasant effects of nicotine to disappear, to be replaced by dependence.

For the established smoker the habit is pleasurable. This is partly due to the psychopharmacological action of nicotine in the brain. Inhalation of tobacco smoke is a remarkably efficient way of getting nicotine to the brain (Fig. 9.4), the interval between inhalation and effect being about ten seconds. Repetition of this process many times with each cigarette and several hundred times a day ensures regular 'shots' and frequent reinforcement. The immediacy of this 'reward' makes smoking a very effective addictive behaviour and this contrasts starkly with the relative remoteness of the health hazards.

Giving up smoking can cause craving and complex pharmacological withdrawal effects, such as restlessness, irritability, sweating, lack of concentration, tremor, and depression. These withdrawal effects may, to some extent, be relieved by nicotine replacement.

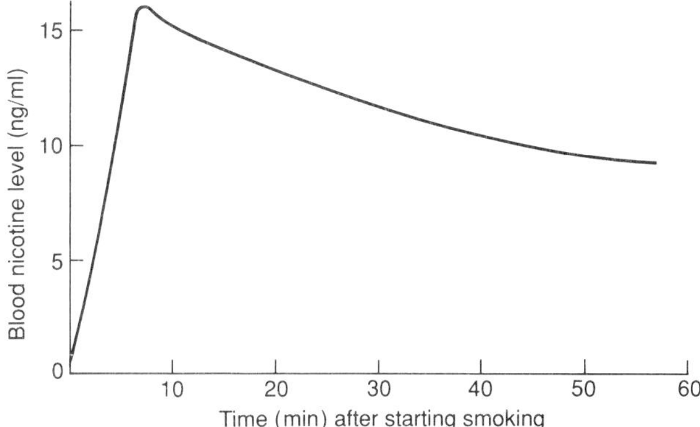

Fig. 9.4 Blood nicotine levels after a single cigarette.

Smoking as a behaviour

But pharmacological addiction to nicotine is not the only or complete explanation for continued smoking. Psychological and social factors also contribute. The habit becomes strongly associated with certain activities and is reinforced by frequent repetition. It may also relieve tension by occupying the hands and mouth in stressful situations.

The rituals of smoking play an important part in maintaining the habit, just as rituals are important in other drug use, including drinking alcohol.

Although the social acceptability of smoking is now declining in Britain and many other countries, acceptance of cigarettes was an act of social intercourse for many years and still is in some places.

Epidemiological studies, first reported in the 1950s by Doll and others, have demonstrated clearly that tobacco smoking greatly increases the risk of lung cancer which is up to 40 times more common in smokers than non-smokers.

Subsequent prospective studies, including a long-term follow-up study of British doctors who were smokers, non-smokers, and ex-smokers, confirmed this and other harmful effects—chiefly on the lungs, heat, and circulation. These studies also showed that stopping smoking is associated with a decline in risk (Figs. 9.5 and 9.6). Cigarette smoking was also shown to be much more dangerous than the smoking of pipes and cigars.

Royal College of Physicians reports

In 1962, the Royal College of Physicians published its first report on 'Smoking and Health'. In this review, the accumulating evidence of harm was

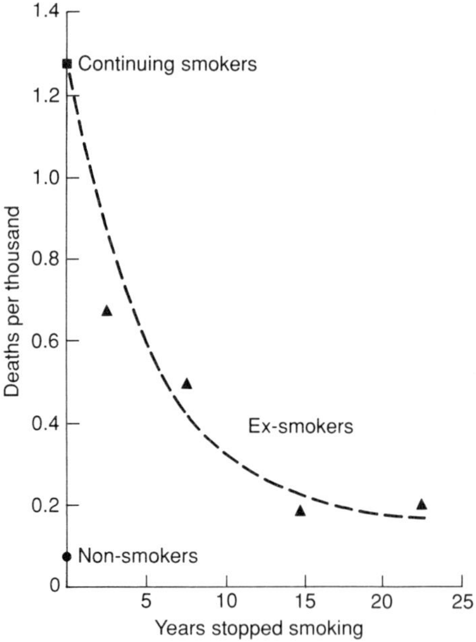

Fig. 9.5 Standardized death rates from lung cancer for cigarette smokers and ex-smokers for various periods and for non-smokers. (From Royal College of Physicians 1971, after Doll and Hill's study of British doctors.)

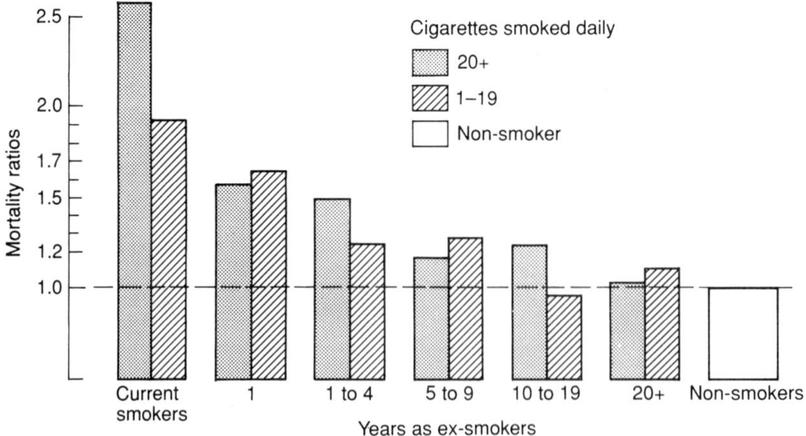

Fig. 9.6 Diminished risk of death from coronary heart disease in former light and heavy smokers. Both light and heavy smokers show a steady decline in risk after stopping until, after 10 to 20 years, it is little different from the risk of non-smokers. (From Royal College of Physicians 1977, after Hammond and Garfinkel.)

examined, and it was concluded that cigarette smoking was the most important contemporary challenge to preventive medicine. It was as important a cause of death as the great epidemics of the past such as cholera, typhoid, and tuberculosis. This report, and subsequent ones, received widespread publicity (see Box 9.1).

Box 9.1: The Royal College of Physicians report on smoking and health (1983)

It is estimated that tobacco smoking accounts annually for:

- 15–20 per cent of all deaths in Britain, i.e. a total of at least 100 000 deaths (25 000 below age 65 years);
- 90 per cent of the 40 000 lung cancer deaths;
- 75 per cent of the 20 000 chronic lung disease deaths;
- 25 per cent of the 180 000 coronary heart disease deaths.

It also contributes to strokes, other vascular deaths, and many cancers.

Size of the smoking risk

About a quarter of all regular smokers are killed early by their smoking (Box 9.2), losing 10–15 years of life on average.

Box 9.2: The risks of smoking in perspective

Peto has provided a graphic illustration of smoking risks:

Of 1000 young men who smoke regularly,

- 1 will be murdered,
- 6 will be killed on the roads,
- 250 will be killed by tobacco.

Interaction with other risks Coronary heart disease is the commonest cause of death in Britain and other developed countries, causing a third of deaths in men (including half of all deaths in middle-aged men) and a quarter of deaths in women.

Smoking increases the risk of coronary heart disease death two- or threefold overall, but as much as tenfold in young men. Alcohol and smoking both cause cancers of the mouth, pharynx, and oesophagus and together act synergistically in doing this. Certain industrial products, notably asbestos, also potentiate the harm of smoking.

Special hazards for women Smoking increases the risk of vascular disease in women on oral contraceptives, at least in older women. It also doubles the risk of carcinoma of the cervix. Women who smoke during pregnancy have an increased risk of miscarriage or of giving birth to smaller babies with an increased perinatal mortality.

Passive smoking

Recent evidence indicates that the harmful effects of smoking are not confined to the smoker. Inhalation of 'side-stream' smoke can cause disease in non-smokers. There is evidence that:

- young children whose parents smoke have twice as many chest infections as others;
- non-smokers working in smoky environments have impaired lung function;
- non-smoking wives of husbands who smoke have an increased risk of lung cancer.

It is estimated that about 300 lung cancer deaths in non-smokers can actually be attributed to passive smoking—as can a significant, though less easily estimated, number of coronary heart disease deaths. There is increasingly acknowledgement of the rights of non-smokers. Restrictions on smoking in public places are increasing, are in line with public attitudes, and are largely respected.

Understanding smokers' attitudes and beliefs

Adoption of smoking in childhood or adolescence is largely a social process. It then becomes an established habit which confers psychological benefits, some attributable to nicotine to which dependence develops.

For health reasons, but also because of financial costs and increasing social pressures, the majority of smokers report that they want to stop smoking. Surveys show that about:

- three quarters of smokers have at some time tried to give up;
- half of smokers have made at least three attempts to stop.

Although 90 per cent of smokers acknowledge the health risks of smoking, most believe the risks are confined to 'heavy' smokers. Many regard smoking less than 20 cigarettes daily as relatively safe and the majority do not think that the kind of smoking they do is all that harmful or that they would do themselves much good by giving up. They underestimate the harmful effect of moderate smoking and set the 'abuse level' above their own consumption.

A common view is that 'any harm done is already done'. Generally, although smokers accept the increased risk of bronchitis as common, they believe the risk of lung cancer or heart disease is small and that stopping smoking will not help.

'Stress' is the usual reason given for continued smoking. The majority of smokers say that they would make a serious attempt to stop if their doctors advised them to do so. Only about a third say that they have ever received such advice.

Helping smokers to stop

There is no 'magic cure' or single prescription for stopping smoking. Successful ex-smokers report an infinite variety of successful methods. *Stages* in the progress from being a smoker to becoming an ex-smoker are:

1. thinking about stopping;
2. preparing to stop;
3. actually stopping;
4. staying stopped.

'External influences' include: cigarette tax; advertising bans; and social pressures.

The role of primary health care: giving advice

Health professionals, especially doctors and nurses in general practice, are of key importance in helping patients to stop smoking, and research has confirmed this. Media campaigns have been shown only to motivate smokers to stop rather than to help them to do so. Simple advice from a general practitioner, even given on just one occasion, can achieve a long-term cessation rate of about 5 per cent, roughly doubling the 'natural' cessation rate.

Self-help leaflets have been shown to enhance the effect of verbal advice and some studies have demonstrated that more intensive advice and frequent follow-up can achieve cessation rates of up to 20 per cent (though the practical feasibility of this is questionable).

In specialist smoking cessation clinics also, higher success rates have been reported; but such clinics recruit more motivated patients than the average and provide a good deal of support.

The *principles* of giving advice on stopping smoking are shown in Box 9.3.

Raising the issue

There is increasing evidence that patients expect doctors to ask them about aspects of lifestyle, especially smoking, and such enquiry and advice is part of

Box 9.3: The principle of giving advice on stopping smoking

1. Raise the issue.
2. Record smoking habits in medical records.
3. Enquire about interest in giving up.
4. Give information and advice on how to stop.
5. Help plan a strategy for giving up.
6. Offer follow-up and support.
7. Help non-smokers and ex-smokers not to start.

the 1990 NHS general practice contract. Many patients welcome enquiry, advice, and help.

Given the importance of smoking as a cause of ill-health, doctors should routinely ask patients whether they smoke and give advice. Enquiry indicates to the patient the health significance of the habit. Questions should include the numbers of cigarettes smoked and the duration of smoking.

Enquiry about smoking should certainly be an essential part of any consultation with a patient who has smoking-related diseases, diabetes mellitus, hypertension, or forthcoming operations. It is also essential to ask women who take oral contraception or are pregnant. In young children with respiratory diseases, parental smoking may be relevant.

Putting smoking '*on the agenda*' in this way provokes 'thinking about stopping', establishes and reinforces motivation, and encourages a review of the reasons for stopping. The *most important* reasons are the individual's own reasons and the positive gains.

Recording smoking habits

As the most important cause of preventable disease and premature death, smoking habit warrants recording in medical records. However, surveys of such records generally show that only a small minority contain information about smoking habit .This can be greatly improved by systematic enquiry and recording. Recording (and retrieval) of such information can be improved by special record cards or sticky labels.

Enquiring about interest in giving up

This is the natural sequel to enquiry about and recording of smoking habit. The majority of smokers express interest in stopping and have tried at least once.

Explore the *smoker's belief* about:

- the effects smoking has on him/her;
- how serious he/she thinks the risk is;

- the perceived benefits of stopping;
- the obstacles to stopping.

Typical questions to ask are shown in Box 9.4.

> **Box 9.4: Some typical questions**
>
> - Do you think smoking affects people's health?
> - Does smoking affect *your* health?
> - Does it affect you in other ways?
> - What about your health in the future?
> - What are the chances *your* health might be affected?
> - What would be the main benefits for *you* of stopping smoking?
> - What things prevent you from stopping smoking?

Giving information and advice on how to stop

In spite of the widespread assumption that there can be few who remain ignorant of the facts, information about the health hazards of smoking, with emphasis on the benefits of stopping, remains important. Misconceptions about the risks of smoking and benefits of stopping should be corrected. False beliefs about danger being confined to heavy smokers are especially prevalent.

Information personally relevant to the individual is more important than general facts, and specific and concrete facts are preferable to vague generalizations. Firm, sympathetic advice to stop should be offered. Failure to offer such advice maybe interpreted as tacit approval of continuance.

Mass media information and programmes, including television, radio, newspapers, and public campaigns, provide important 'agenda-setting' information.

Increasing motivation Although most ex-smokers achieved success 'on their own', others need help. Reseach has shown that doctors and nurses in primary care can be effective in helping smokers to stop.

Health and money seem to be the key concerns influencing attitudes to stopping smoking. The health benefits of giving up, when accepted, produce the most committed response.

Intention to stop may be provoked by changes in belief or perceptions, such as:

- the consequences if smoking continues;
- the consequences of stopping;
- the importance of what may happen after continuing or stopping.

Positive attitudes to giving up will provoke desire to do so—and maybe the intention and resolve to stop. An 'intender' becomes a 'trier' and attempts to stop. Some attempts succeed—not necessarily the first time—and the chances of success are enhanced by confidence in the ability to succeed.

Helping plan a strategy for giving up

Stopping completely rather than gradually cutting down is generally best, but cutting out 'less essential' cigarettes first may sometimes be helpful.

Putting into practice previously planned preparations needs encouragement. Review of the reasons for stopping may reinforce determination.

Self-help leaflets supplement verbal advice, act as a reminder, and are a source of reference. Other useful adjuncts may be use of a CO monitor or the prescription of nicotine chewing gum (see below). Selfmonitoring with a simple diary may help. 'Self-rewards', such as treats, presents, or putting money saved in a conspicuous place, may also be helpful.

Planning how to cope with 'smoking situations' and 'danger times', such as tea breaks, and after meals, when having a drink is important. Alternative ways of relaxing may need to be learned, such as going for a walk, deep breathing exercises, and yoga. Involvement of a spouse or close friend can increase commitment.

Choosing a '*stopping day*', although difficult, is important and may be:

- a little ahead;
- at a relatively stress-free time;
- at a time of change in routine, e.g. holiday;
- New Year, National No Smoking Day, birthday, or any other event.

For some, stopping may be provoked suddenly by personal illness or smoking-related illness or death in a relative or friend.

Offering follow-up and support

A 'warning' of follow-up may be a stimulus to action and perseverance. Follow-up and support can also be an important encouragement. Research has shown that sustained follow-up and support can achieve higher success rates in smoking cessation.

Weight gain occurs in some patients but it is often temporary and should be managed by reassurance and if necessary by dietary advice later.

Staying stopped

Staying stopped is generally the most difficult stage. Vigilance is essential as excuses to restart easily spring to mind. Avoidance of the 'Just one cigarette wouldn't hurt' temptation is essential. The support of others at this time may be especially valuable.

Helping non-smokers and ex-smokers not to start

Opportunities to reinforce the benefits of non-smoking should be utilized. Asking known non-smokers and ex-smokers about their smoking status will emphasize the health importance of the habit.

Helping those who can't stop with advice alone

Most of those who stop smoking do so 'on their own'. Others will be helped by simple advice as discussed above. But for some, additional measures may be helpful.

Prescribing nicotine chewing gum

Some patients find nicotine chewing gum helpful in giving up smoking, particular in coping with withdrawal symtoms. However, it is an adjunct to advice, not a 'magic cure'.

Research has demonstrated the efficacy of nicotine gum but its effectiveness depends on careful instruction and proper use. It offers a substitute source of nicotine, allowing the smoker to cope with the problems of breaking the habit before also having to deal with nicotine withdrawal, so that craving is reduced. The 4 mg strength is currently available on prescription only (but not in the NHS) as Nicorette. The 2 mg strength is available from pharmacists, without prescription.

Chewing the gum releases the nicotine which is absorbed through the lining of the mouth. Each piece should be chewed slowly and intermittently for about thirty minutes. Incorrect chewing technique may result in soreness of the mouth or throat, hiccups, or indigestion.

If found helpful, its use should continue for three or four months.

It should not be used in pregnancy, by nursing mothers, or by those with peptic ulcers.

Smokers' clinics

Smokers' clinics have a limited role in smoking cessation. They are a specialist rather than front-line service and are relatively few in number. Their functional principles are largely those of group therapy.

Nicotine chewing gum has been shown to be particularly effective in the context of such clinics, probably because of the high level of motivation of participants, careful instruction in and supervision of its use, persistence, and the high level of continuing support.

Other methods

Nicotine skin patches, as a new method of nicotine replacement, are currently being tested and early results look promising.

Several other methods, such as acupuncture, hypnosis, special antismoking aids, and five-day plan courses, are available. Some smokers find them helpful but none has been shown by scientific evaluation to have a specific effect.

No smoker should be discouraged from trying a method he/she wishes to try as long as it is safe. Exaggerated claims for unproven methods may reduce credibility and be counterproductive.

Organization and equipment in the practice

Objectives

1. Smoking status of all patients should be recorded in the medical records in such a way as to be clearly available whenever the patient is seen.
2. Opportunities for doctors and nurses to give information and advice about stopping smoking to those who smoke should be sought and used.
3. Practice premises should be a smoke-free environment.

Record audit

Reviewing records is a useful way of measuring achievement and stimulating improvement. A random sample of records can be scanned for any information about whether the patient smokes or not. Generally, less than 20 per cent of records contain such information. A reasonable initial target is to achieve such recordings in 50 per cent of notes.

Equipment and leaflets

The most important thing is simple advice. But leaflets are a useful aid and the practice should have a stock of these readily available (see addresses).

A CO monitor may be a useful educational instrument because levels of carbon monoxide in expired breath correlate closely with blood levels of carboxyhaemoglobin. Non-smokers can have a level of CO up to 10 parts per million, but smokers can have levels of 50 parts per million or more and such levels remain raised for several hours after smoking (Fig. 9.7).

Measurement of expired CO with a small, portable monitor may potentiate the effect of advice in helping patients to stop smoking. It may also be used to validate self-reports of smoking cessation.

Public health policy and political action

Doctors have a role in regard to smoking not only with individual patients but also in contributing to public health policy and political action.

Measures which should be adopted include:

- abolition of all forms of promotion of tobacco products;
- raising price through taxation;

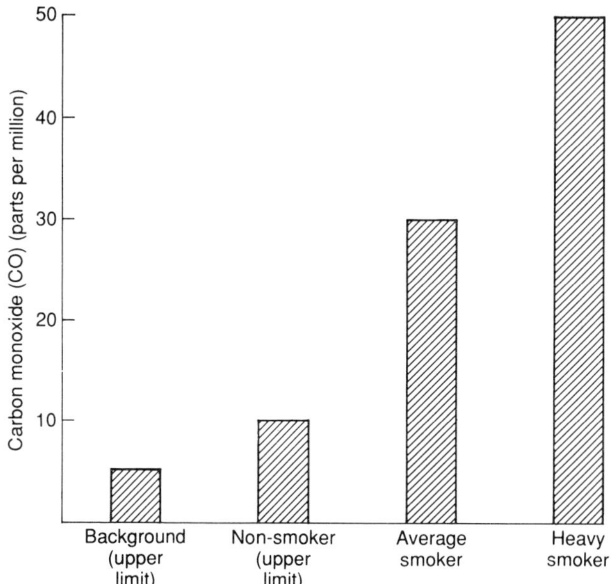

Fig. 9.7 CO levels in non-smokers' and smokers' breath (and environmental CO level).

- prominent explicit health warnings on cigarette packets;
- public information and education programmes;
- effective banning of sales to children;
- reducing the tar content of cigarettes;
- controlling smoking in public places and workplaces.

Legislation is required to implement most of these measures; voluntary agreements have limited usefulness.

Through medical organizations and by direct communication with Government ministers and Members of Parliament, doctors can assist adoption of these measures.

Summary

- Cigarette consumption is declining but smoking is three times as common in manual workers as professional men.
- Smoking causes over 100 000 deaths each year in Britain—mainly from lung cancer, coronary heart disease, and obstructive lung disease.
- Passive smoking also causes disease in non-smokers and is responsible for about 300 lung cancer deaths annually in non-smokers.

- Doctors in primary care can help smokers to stop smoking and have an important role in smoking cessation.
- Patients should routinely be asked and advised about smoking.
- Verbal advice should be supplemented with a patient leaflet.
- Adjuncts to advice include nicotine chewing gum.
- Doctors have a political role in relation to tobacco control.

Addresses (for information and leaflets)

Action on Smoking and Health (ASH)
109 Gloucester Place
Telephone London W1H 3PH
071–935–3519

Health Education Authority
Hamilton House
Mabledon Place
London WC1H 9TX
Telephone 071–631–0930

Scottish Committee
Action on Smoking and Health
6 Castle Street
Edinburgh EH2 3AT
Telephone 031–225–4725

Scottish Health Education Group
Woodburn House
Canaan Lane
Edinburgh EH10 4SG
Telephone 031–447–8044

Heartbeat Wales/Welsh Promotion Authority
24 Park Place
Cardiff CF1 3BA
Telephone 0222–378855

Ulster Cancer Foundation/ASH Northern Ireland
40–42 Eglantine Avenue
Belfast BT9 6TX
Telephone 0232–663281

Further reading

Ashton, R. and Stepney, R. (1982). *Smoking: psychology and pharmacology.* Tavistock, London.
British Medical Association and Imperial Cancer Research Fund (1988). *Help your patient stop.* BMA, London.
Kottke, T. E., Battista, R. N., and DeFriese, G. H. (1988). Attributes of successful smoking cessation interventions in medical practice: a meta-analysis of 39 controlled trials. *Journal of the American Medical Association*, **259**, 2883–9.
Marsh, A. and Matheson, J. (1983). Smoking attitudes and behaviour. HMSO, London.
OPCS (1990). OPCS Monitor SS90/2, 4 April 1990.
Royal College of Physicians (1971). *Smoking and health now: a new report and summary on smoking and its effects on health.* Pitman, London.
Royal College of Physicians (1977). *Smoking or health: the third report from the Royal College of Physicians, London.* Pitman, London.
Royal College of Physicians (1983). *Health or smoking? Follow-up report of the Royal College of Physicians.* Pitman, London.
UICO (1984). *Guidelines to Smoking Cessation*, UICC technical report series No. 79. International Union Against Cancer, Geneva. 1984.
World Health Organization (1979). *Technical report series* No. 636. WHO, Geneva.
World Health Organization (1979). *Controlling the smoking epidemic*, Report of WHO Expert Committee on smoking control. WHO, Geneva.

10 Healthy eating

Godfrey Fowler

Diet and health

For most of their existence human beings have been hunter-gatherers. During that time our diet was very different from that now eaten in developed countries. There has therefore been considerable adaptation to dietary change.

In Britain, it seems that the population was relatively well nourished until the Industrial Revolution. Then industralization contribued to wide variation in food intake between rich and poor. Nutritional deficiencies amongst the poor became common. Undernutrition and nutritional deficiencies remained a significant problem in Britain until World War II. Then improvements in agricultural techniques and the more even distribution of an adequate diet substantially reduced dietary deficiencies.

Since the 1950s, the nutritional problem affecting the majority of the population in Britain and other developed countries has been the excessive consumption of food, particularly of certain types. 'Overnutrition' rather than 'undernutrition' now therefore poses the major dietary threat to health in developed countries. This overnutrition results in excessive calorie consumption and the most important contributor is fat which provides 42 per cent of calorie intake in the average British diet. Ironically, in much of the Third World, starvation, undernutrition, and deficiencies of essential nutrients remain major problems contributing to much ill-health and premature death.

Diseases of affluence

A variety of diseases that have become common in developed countries but remain rare in developing ones are sometimes referred to as 'diseases of affluence'. However, in developing countries, these diseases are also beginning to affect the richer sections of the population, and they seem to be attributable, to some extent at least, to aspects of a so-called 'Western diet'. These 'diseases of affluence' are listed in Box 10.1.

Box 10.1: Some diseases of affluence

Obesity
Coronary heart disease
Hypertension
Diabetes mellitus (type II (NIDDM)
Dental caries
Various cancers
Large bowel disorders
Gallstones
Haemorrhoids and varicose veins

Western diet

A Western diet is characterized by a preponderance of foods with:

- a high content of fat (especially 'saturated' fat);
- a high content of refined carbohydrate (sugar);
- a low content of ('fibre').

These shifts to a higher fat and sugar content and a lower fibre content in the diet have been a twentieth-century phenomenon. There has also been an increase in salt (sodium) intake and alcohol consumption has also increased rapidly in recent years.

Many foods are 'processed' so that identification of ingredients is difficult, and total energy (calorie) intake is now generally in excess of needs, especially as average energy expenditure has declined because work is generally less strenuous.

Obesity

Apart from being a cosmetic or social problem, obesity may also impair health. If an individual is above (or below) the range of weights for a given height, the risk of illness and mortality increases. This is a fact well known to insurance companies (Fig. 10.1). Being overweight is associated with increased risk of coronary heart disease, hypertension, stroke, diabetes, gall-bladder diseases, some cancers, post-operative complications, and accidents. For a given height there is therefore a desirable weight, i.e. that associated with the lowest mortality risk. The relationship between weight and height is best demonstrated by the body mass index (BMI) as described in Box 10.2. The relationship of weight to height, defining the desirable range and grades of obesity, is illustrated in Fig. 10.2.

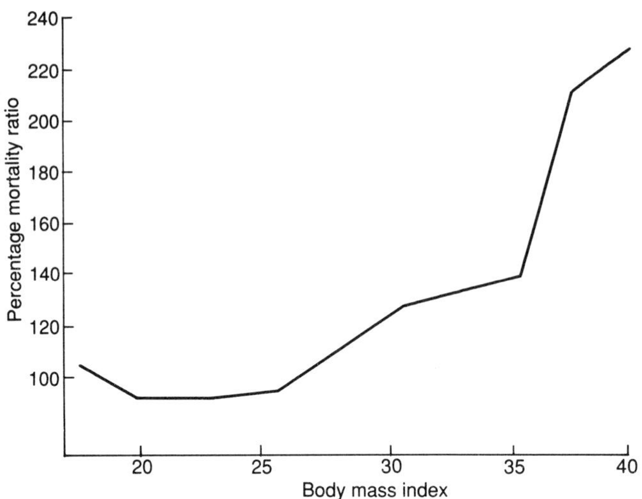

Fig. 10.1 Mortality in relation to body weight for men aged 15–39 years. (From Royal College of Physicians 1983)

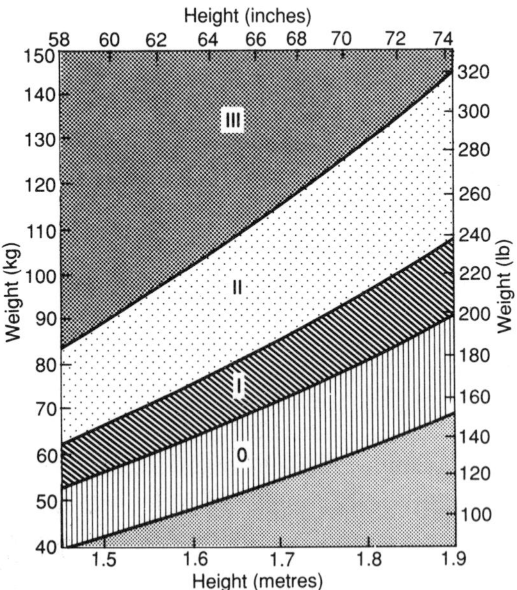

Fig. 10.2 Relationship of weight to height, defining the desirable range (0), and grades I, II, and III (obesity). (From Garrow 1988)

Box 10.2: The body mass index

A convenient index of relative weight is the *body mass index* (BMI) or Quetelet's index. This is weight (kilograms) divided by the square of the height (metres)

$$\text{BMI} = \frac{\text{weight (kg)}}{\text{height}^2\ (\text{M}^2)}.$$

Adult 'desirable' or 'acceptable' weight corresponds to a BMI of 20–25.

Obesity is usually defined as weight which is 20 per cent or more above the upper limit of 'desirable' weight and corresponds to a BMI of 30 or more.

Almost 10 per cent of the adult population is obese by this definition and about one-third is *overweight*, i.e. has a BMI > 25.

Obesity occurs when energy intake exceeds expenditure. Control of obesity generally involves reduction of calorie intake and increase in energy expenditure.

Coronary heart disease

Coronary heart disease is multifactorial in origin but diet is the key environmental factor, and the relationship between diet and coronary heart disease has provoked intensive study over several decades. In one of the first and best-known investigations, a prospective study started in the 1950s, Keys showed a relationship between coronary heart disease mortality rates and the percentage of calories derived from dietary saturated fat in cohorts from various countries (Fig. 10.3).

In later studies, it was found that those moving from a country with a low average saturated fat consumption and low coronary heart disease rate to one with a high consumption and high coronary heart disease rate tended, in time, to acquire the coronary heart disease rate of the adoptive country. For example, Japanese people moving to California, in due course, developed the disease.

It has since been demonstrated in many studies that populations with the diets low in saturated fat and with a high ratio of polyunsaturated to saturated fat have a low incidence of coronary heart disease and conversely that a high saturated fat intake and low polyunsaturated/saturated ratio is associated with a high incidence of coronary heart disease.

Within a given population, there is less conclusive evidence of the relationship between diet and coronary heart disease, but there is a strong link

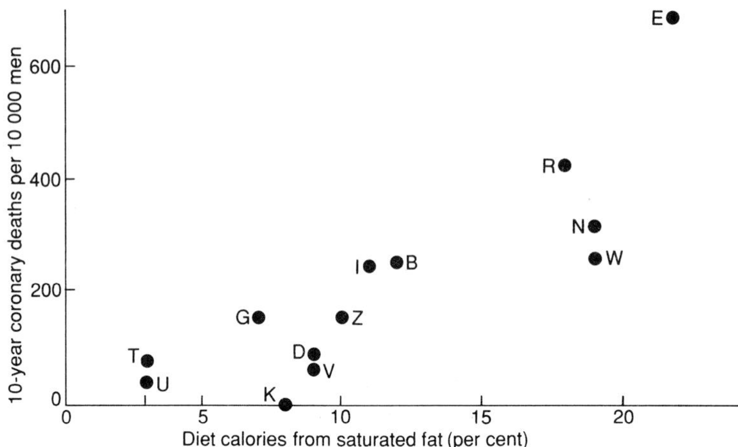

Fig. 10.3 Relationship between the dietary fat in different countries and coronary heart disease death rates. The relationship of the median plasma cholesterol level to 10-year CHD mortality in 16 male cohorts of the seven countries study. B = Belgrade (Yugoslavia); D = Dalmatia (Yugoslavia); E = east Finland; G = Corfu; I = Italian railroad; K = Crete; N = Zutphen (Nehterlands); T = Tanushimaru (Japan); R = American railroad; U = Ushibuka (Japan; V = Velike Krsna (Yugoslavia); W = West Finland; Z = Zrenjanin (Yugoslavia). (From Keys 1980)

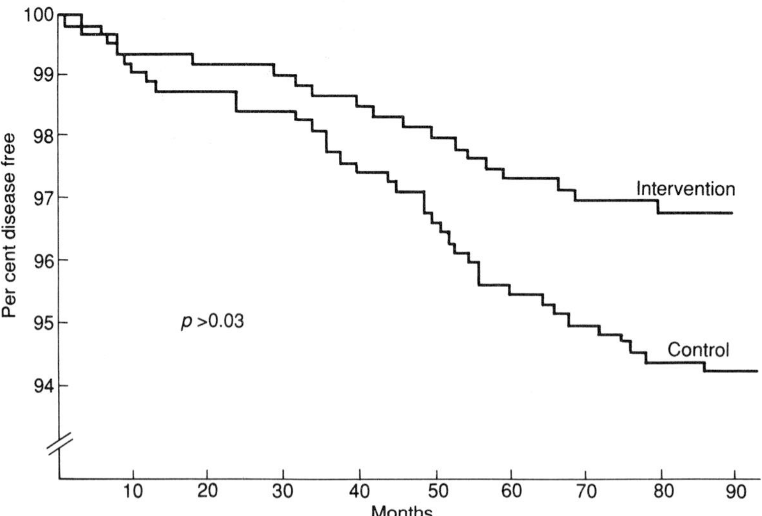

Fig. 10.4 Life-table analysis of CHD (fatal and non-fatal myocardial infarction and sudden death) in intervention and control groups (the Oslo study). (From Hjermann *et al.* 1981)

between the mean population blood level of cholesterol (especially LDL cholesterol) and coronary heart disease incidence, and experimental studies in animals have demonstrated that high-fat diets can cause atherosclerotic lesions.

There is evidence from dietary intervention trials (e.g. the Oslo study illustrated in Fig. 10.4) that reducing saturated fat intake can reduce coronary heart disease incidence and mortality, and that reduction of plasma cholesterol levels in man by drugs and/or diet may be associated with reversal of atheroma.

The basic features of the relationships between dietary fat and coronary heart disease are listed in Box 10.3.

Box 10.3: Features of the relationship between dietary fat and coronary heart disease

- Accumulating evidence indicates that the relationship of dietary fat to coronary heart disease is not simply that of a positive link with saturated fats.
- Unsaturated fats (and particularly linoleic acid) may have a protective effect.
- The ratio of polyunsaturated to saturated fats is probably as important as total fat consumption.
- Dietary cholesterol is probably less important than is generally thought. It has only a small effect on plasma cholesterol compared with saturated fats. Many people confuse dietary with blood cholesterol.

It has been shown in many prospective studies that plasma total (and LDL) cholesterol is a major risk factor for coronary heart disease. The major dietary influence on total (and LDL) cholesterol is the amount and type of fat consumed. Saturated fatty acids have an elevating effect and polyunsaturated fats tend to lower total and LDL cholesterol. Blood cholesterol levels in people on different diets are illustrated in Fig. 10.5 As well as their effect on lipids (and hence atheroma) dietary fats also influence thrombosis. Certain polyunsaturated fatty acids (e.g. eicosapentaenoic acid) which are found in oily fish are potent inhibitors of thrombosis (acting as competitive antagonists of thromboxane A). Other polyunsaturated fats found in seed oils (e.g. linoleic acid) have a small inhibitory effect.

Hypertension

Although hypertension is multifactorial, in studies of populations a correlation between the incidence of hypertension and average daily salt intake has

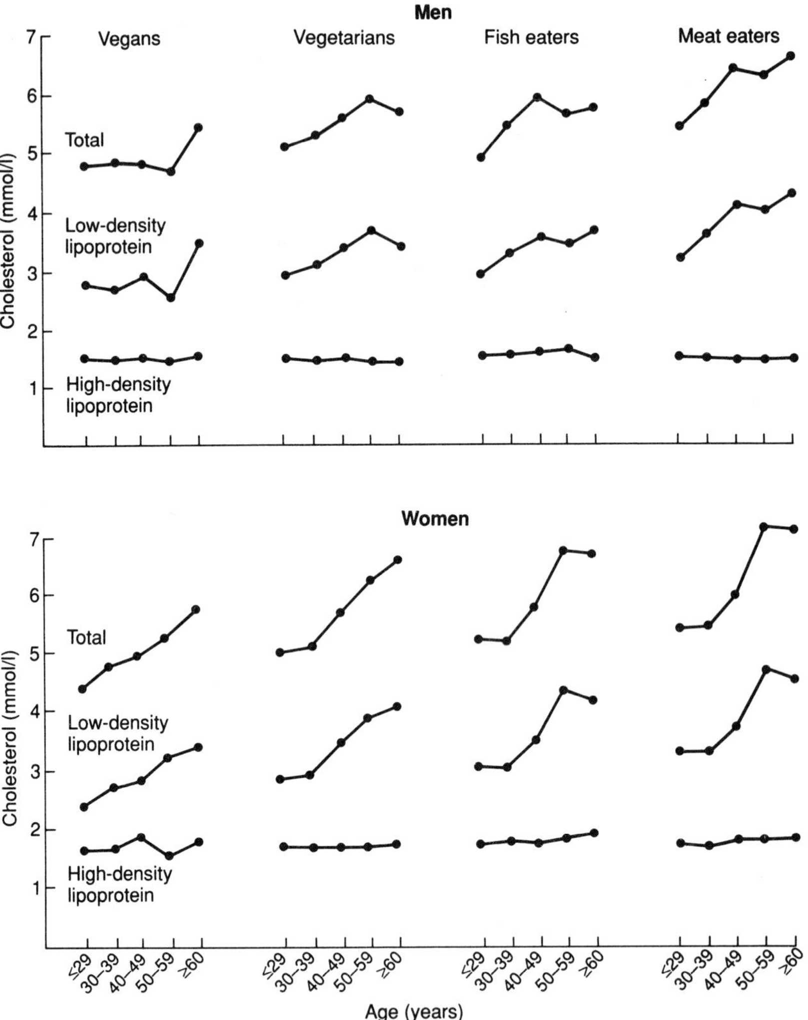

Fig. 10.5 Plasma cholesterol concentration and dietary habits. (From Thorogood *et al.* 1987)

been found. In remote Pacific islanders with salt intakes of less than 2 g a day hypertension is rare. In northern Japan, where the population has an average salt intake greater than 25 g daily, hypertension and stroke are common. However, the correlation between salt intake and hypertension in individuals is not clearly demonstrable, although a reduction in sodium intake can lower blood pressure. There appears to be much individual variation in susceptibility to sodium.

10.4: The relationship between alcohol consumption and coronary heat disease

- Alcohol consumption within populations is positively correlated with hypertension and coronary heart disease, and reduction of alcohol intake in individuals can contribute to hypertension control.
- Obesity is strongly related to hypertension and weight loss can lower blood pressure.

There is an important relationship between alcohol consumption and coronary heart disease (see Box 10.4).

Diabetes

The association of diabetes with obesity has been recognized for a long time. Non-insulin-dependent type II (maturity onset) diabetes is highly correlated with obesity but insulin-dependent type I (juvenile) diabetes is not.

This link between the prevalence of type II diabetes and obesity is apparent when the prevalence of obesity and diabetes in different countries is studied and also when the relationship between obesity and diabetes in a given population is investigated.

Although there is a popular misconception that eating too much sugar causes diabetes it is excessive energy intake, usually from a high fat consumption, which contributes to obesity and may, in turn, cause diabetes.

Dietary fibre may have a protective effect. When comparing different populations and different individuals diabetes is less common in those with a high fibre intake. Diet is important in the management of both type I and type II diabetes and diets high in fibre-rich carbohydrates improve diabetic control.

Dental caries

Dental caries is tooth decay due to cavitation and erosion of enamel. This is caused by the action of acids arising from bacterial fermentation of sugars in the mouth. In countries where unrefined foods form the bulk of the diet, caries is rare; but the addition of sugar and other refined foods to the diet rapidly increases the incidence.

Frequency of consumption of sugary foods, especially between meals, is probably as important as total consumption.

Although dental health in Britain is poor, there has been an improvement in recent years. This is probably partly related to reduced average sugar consumption but more importantly to fluoridation of water in many places.

Addition of fluoride to water in a concentration of one part per million enables an intake of fluoride sufficient to increase enamel resistance to caries.

Cancer

Suggestions of a relationship between diet and cancer have a long history. Real interest in diet and cancer developed in the 1960s when studies showed that the geographical variation in the incidenced of some cancers correlated with patterns of food intake.

In a recent review, Doll and Peto estimated that about one third of all cancers may be attributable to aspects of diet (although much of the evidence is tentative). This is about the same proportion of cancers as are caused by smoking. Studies of the relationship between food intake and disease are difficult to perform because of the problems of accurate dietary assessment and measurement.

Cancer of the large bowel is the second commonest cause of death from cancer in Britain (after lung cancer in men and breast cancer in women). It is about ten times more common in Western countries than inthe Third World. In epidemiological studies, the incidence of bowel cancer has been shown to be positively correlated with fat and meat intake, and negatively correlated with dietary fibre, fruit, and vegetable intake. The results of epidemiological studies also suggest dietary factors contribute to cancers of the oesophagus, stomach, liver, and pancreas. Breast cancer incidence in populations shows a strong positive correlation with fat intake. There may also be an independent association between obesity and breast cancer incidence (See Box 10.5).

Box 10.5: The relationship between diet and cancer

- Causative factors appear to be obesity, fat intake, meat consumption, and alcohol intake.
- Protective factors appear to be dietary fibre, fruit, and vegetable intake.

Large bowel disorders

Various chronic bowel disorders including constipation, irritable bowel syndrome, and colonic diverticulosis occur more commonly in those eating a Western diet than in those countries where a basically vegetarian, high-fibre diet is normal.

Studies of vegetarians show they are much less prone to these conditions than non-vegetarians. Bowel transit time is inversely correlated with dietary fibre intake and this may be part of the explanation. However, no formal intervention studies have shown a protective effect of dietary fibre against bowel disorders.

Other diseases

Among other diseases common in developed countries and rare in the developing ones are gallstones, appendicitis, haemorrhoids, and varicose veins. There is some evidence that dietary factors may contribute to these.

Gallstones are associated with obesity and lower dietary fibre intake. Appendicitis rates are not only high in countries in which the population has low average dietary fibre intake but, within populations, rates seem inversely correlated with dietary fibre.

There is increasing concern about alcohol as a cause of ill-health and premature death in Britain. This is discussed in Chapter 11.

Dietary recommendations

As has been indicated, a Western diet appears to contribute to many 'modern' diseases. In concert with this increasing public awareness, there is interest in modifying diet to reduce the risk of these diseases and a desire for advice about a 'healthy diet'. However, owing to the uncertainty about the relationship between diet and disease, some aspects of dietary advice remain controversial. Despite this, there is now a broad consensus among experts about the essential features of such a diet for the adult population.

Dietary guidelines have been agreed in the UK which are consistent with those in other developed countries such as the USA, Canada, the Scandinavian countries, Australia, and New Zealand.

Desirable body weight

Overweight and obesity arise from an excess of energy intake over expenditure. Energy requirements vary greatly among individuals, and achieving and maintaining a balance depend on hereditary, psychological, and physiological factors. The mechanism is imperfectly understood. In most cases, the basic problem is that energy (calorie) intake is in excess of daily requirement. A sedentary occupation and lifestyle with relatively little physical activity are often contributory factors.

The first priority is to achieve and maintain 'desirable' or 'acceptable' body weight, i.e. a body mass index (BMI) of 20–25 (see p. 125). Guidelines for achieving weight control are shown in Box 10.6. Reduction in fat, sugars, and other refined carbohydrates in the diet is the most effective way of reducing calorie intake. Complex carbohydrates (whole-grain bread, cereals, vegetables, and fruit) can be substituted. Alcohol may be an important source

Box 10.6: Guidelines for achieving weight control

Weight control can be aided by:

- an awareness of food eaten, especially regarding its fat content;
- a modification of diet, if necessary, along the lines indicated above;
- an avoidance of eating between meals, especially high-energy food such as crisps and biscuits;
- regular weighing;
- regular exercise, e.g. walking;
- suitable motivation to control weight.

of calories and will therefore need careful control. Substitution of unprocessed foods for processed foods is likely to reduce energy intake.

Appropriate labelling of food would improve education about composition of foods, particularly with respect to their fat content.

Reducing the risk of coronary heart disease

The major concern about diet in Britain and other developed countries is its relationship to coronary heart disease—a major killer.

Although there are still areas of dispute, there is now substantial agreement on the basic recommendations for dietary change to reduce risk of coronary heart disease. These recommendations need to be implemented in childhood (but not infancy) and early adult life if maximum benefit is to be achieved. For Britain the most recent and authorative guidelines are those arising from the COMA (DHSS Committee on Medical Aspects of Food Policy) Recommendations on Diet in Relation to Cardiovascular Disease (see Box 10.7).

In the average British diet about:

- one-third of fat comes from dairy products'
- one-quarter of fat comes from meat products;
- one-quarter of fat comes from margarine, cooking fats and oils;
- one-sixth of fat comes from crisps, chocolates, cakes, biscuits, etc.

Saturated fats are in meat, dairy produce, hard margarines, sauces, puddings, and some vegetable fats (e.g. coconut and palm oil). Polyunsaturated fats are in some vegetable oils (sunflower, corn, and soya oils), in soft margarine (high in polyunsaturates), in nuts, and in oily fish such as herring, mackerel, and trout. Implementation of the COMA recommendations can be facilitated by following the guidelines in Box 10.8.

Box 10.7: COMA recommendations

The essential features of these *recommendations* are as follows:

- The total fat intake should be reduced to 35 per cent of food energy, representing about 80 g/day (the present average level is 42 per cent, representing over 100 g/day).
- Saturated fat intake should be no more than 15 per cent of food energy (present level about 20 per cent).
- The ratio of polyunsaturated to saturated fats should be increased to about 0.45 (present level about 0.23).
- Fibre-rich carbohydrates (bread, cereals, fruit, and vegetables) should be increased to compensate for reduced fat intake.

Box 10.8: Practical dietary advice

Implementation of the COMA recommendations can be facilitated by substituting:

- semi-skimmed or skimmed milk for ordinary milk;
- soft margarine high in polysaturates for butter or hard margarines;
- low-fat yoghourt for cream;
- low-fat cheeses (cottage cheese, Edam, Camembert) for high-fat cheeses (Cheddar, Stilton);
- chicken or fish more often for red meat.

Fruit and vegetables

There has recently been much interest in the role of high fruit and vegetable intake in providing anti-oxidant vitamin C, E, and beta-carotene. Anti-oxidants appear to inhibit the action of free radicals on cholesterol—an action which potentiates the atherogenic action of cholesterol. High fruit and vegetable intakes may be one factor in Mediterranean diets contributing to the relatively low incidence of coronary heart disease.

The role of primary health care

There is evidence that patients expect their doctors to be interested in aspects of lifestyle, including diet and weight. Some useful questions to ask patients about their diet are shown in Box 10.9.

Box 10.9: Some useful questions about diet

The following questions can act as a stimulus for discussion about diet.

1. What sort of milk do you usually have?
2. What sort of bread do you usually eat?
3. What sort of fat or oil do you use for cooking?
4. Do you put butter or margarine on bread?
5. How often do you eat fresh fruit?
6. How often do you eat fresh green vegetables?
7. How often do you eat fresh fish?
8. Do you have sugar in tea/coffee?
9. How often do you eat sweets/chocolate?
10. Do you usually read food labels?

Simple information, advice and support may be more useful than more complex approaches which may lead to confusion. Advice should be tailored to the needs of the individual as much as possible. Practice nurses have a particularly important role to play in giving advice about diet. Verbal advice should be supplemented with simple leaflets. These should emphasize basic issues and be well illustrated.

Dieticians clearly have an important part to play but more in educating doctors and nurses than in advizing individual patients. There are too few dieticians, and other health professionals must act as intermediaries. Group support along the lines of 'Weight Watchers' may be found helpful by some. However, unlike advice to stop smoking, the effectiveness of dietary advice in primary care remains to be properly evaluated.

Summary

- Overnutrition, rather than undernutrition, poses a major threat to health in developed countries.
- Excess calorie intake associated with a high consumption of saturated fat is the basis of this overnutrition.
- Coronary heart disease and type II diabetes are substantially attributable to this overnutrition.
- The essential features of dietary recommendations are to reduce total fat intake and substitute polyunsaturated and monounsaturated fats for saturated fats to some degree, to increase fibre-rich carbohydrates, and to ensure a sufficiency of fresh fruit or vegetables.
- As in other aspects of lifestyle, primary care has an important role in giving advice.

References and further reading

Diet and cardiovascular disease (1984). Report of DHSS Committee on Medical Aspects of Food Policy. HMSO, London.

Diet, nutrition and health (1986). Report of the Board of Science and Education. BMA, London.

Doll, R. and Peto, R. (1982). *The causes of cancer*. Oxford University Press.

Garrow, J. (1988). *Obesity and related diseases.* Churchill Livingstone, London.

Hjermann, I., Holme, I., Velve Byre, K., and Leren, P. (1981). *The Lancet*, **ii**, 1303–10.

Keys, A. (1980). *Seven countries. A multiariate analysis of death and coronary heart disease.* Harvard University Press, Cambridge, MA.

Royal College of Physicians (1980). *Medical aspects of dietary fibre*, Royal College of Physicians report. RCP, London.

Royal College of Physicians (1983). *Obesity, Report of the Royal College of Physicians, London.* RCP, London.

Thorogood, M., Carter, R., Benfield, L., McPherson, K., and Mann, J.I. (1987). *British Medical Journal*, **295**, 351–4.

Useful addresses

The Health Education Authority
Hamilton House
Mabledon Place
London WC1H 9TX
(from whom 'Guide to Healthy Eating' is available free)

British Heart Foundation
14 Fitzhardinge Street
London W1H 4DH
(from whom 'Food and Your Heart' is available free)

The Flora project for Heart Disease Prevention
24–28 Bloomsbury Way
London WC1A 2PX
(from whom a series of leaflets on prevention of heart disease is obtainable)

11 Reducing alcohol consumption

Peter Anderson

Is drinking an important health issue?

Alcohol misuse is one of Britain's major health and social problems. Some facts about alcohol use are shown in Box 11.1. It causes accidents, at home, on the road, and at work, domestic and street violence, public disturbances, ill-health, and frequent sickness absences (see Box 11.2). Men drinking over 35 units per week and women drinking over 21 units per week have double the risk of liver cirrhosis, cancers of the pharynx, larynx, and oesophagus, high blood pressure, strokes, and sudden death. In addition, women have double the risk of breast cancer (Anderson *et al.* 1991).

Box 11.1: Some facts about alcohol use

- Most cases of ill-health linked to alcohol occur among light and moderate drinkers, even though only a few of them have other alcohol problems. Even a small reduction in the whole population's drinking would create a major improvement.
- The price of alcoholic drinks in this country has been steadily falling: it is now just have over half what it was in the 1950s. Over the same period alcohol consumption has doubled.
- The British public now drinks the equivalent of more than nine pints of beer a week for each individual over the age of 16.
- Young people are the heaviest drinkers—many have accidents or suffer other harm as a result. Road accidents, most due to drink/driving, are now the single largest killer in this group.

Nurses and doctors have to cope with many of the results of excess drinking. Yet alcohol is still not as widely recognized as a factor in ill-health as is smoking.

For many patients, help with cutting down on drinking may be the single most important influence their nurse or doctor will have on their health.

Box 11.2: Alcohol's effects on the public health

Each year excessive drinking plays a part in:

- 1400 deaths on the road (one in three of the total);
- over 8 million days off work;
- one in four emergency hospital admissions;
- nearly 70 per cent of suicides;
- one in three accidents in the home;
- 60 per cent of serious head injuries;
- 17 000 admissions to psychiatric hospitals;
- up to 28 000 deaths in England.

Preventing alcohol problems

The advice in this chapter aims to prevent rather than to treat alcohol problems. The majority of patients at risk because of their drinking are heavy drinkers who have not yet begun to suffer the consequences of excess alcohol assumption. Advice at an early stage could prevent them from becoming a casualty of alcohol misuse in the future. Firm personal advice lasting 10–15 minutes, backed up by a booklet and the clear understanding that their progress is being followed, has been shown in two studies in the United Kingdom to be effective in helping patients who drink heavily cut down on their drinking, by at least one-third (Tables 11.1 and 11.2).

A useful resource to help nurses and doctors in giving advice to patients is the *Cut down on your drinking pack*, produced by the Health Education

Table 11.1 Medical Research Council study: effectiveness of 15 minute advice on alcohol consumption at 12 month follow-up (Wallace *et al.* 1988)

	Alcohol consumption (units/week)	
	Baseline	12 months
Men		
Treatment	62	44 (18)
Control	64	56 (8)
Women		
Treatment	35	24 (11)
Control	37	30 (7)

Table 11.2 Oxford study: effectiveness of 10 minute advice on alcohol consumption at 12 month follow-up (Anderson and Scott, in press; Scott and Anderson 1990)

	Alcohol consumption (units/week)	
	Baseline	12 months
Men		
Treatment	52	36 (16)
Control	53	44 (9)
Women		
Treatment	35	24 (11)
Control	37	27 (10)

Authority. The pack contains a guide for the nurse and doctor, a poster for the surgery, and 25 self-help booklets for patients.

Identification of patients at risk

The first stage is to identify the patients who are at risk because of their drinking. It is possible to do this by using the standard questions shown in Box 11.3. Guidelines for converting alcohol consumption details are shown in Box 11.4.

Why use standard questions? Because they are a proven, simple, and reliable method of finding out how much a patient drinks (Anderson 1989). Simply asking patients 'How much do you drink?' tends to elicit responses, such as 'Not a lot' or 'Just occasionally'. Use of standard questions should lead to a substantial increase in the recognition of heavy drinkers in your practice. Standard questions such as those given in Box 11.3 can be used as part of health checks and can also be used during consultations with selected patients who may be at risk (see Boxes 11.5 and 11.6).

Blood tests such as gamma glutamyl transpepidose can be a useful check if a patient is suspected of being a heavy drinker, but they are expensive and frequently give a negative result even if the patient is drinking excessively. Moreover, a positive result cannot establish how much the patient actually drinks.

Advising your patient

Give firm but friendly advice to cut down. Reassure the patient that you don't think he or she is an 'alcoholic'. But if he or she continues to drink at the current rate, health damage, and work and personal problems, are most likely to develop.

Box 11.3: Totting up consumption

To help you work out the number of units of alcohol that your patient drinks each week, ask the following questions:

- On average, how many days a week do you have an alcoholic drink? ☐
- On average, on a day when you have had an alcoholic drink, how much do you usually have:

  half pints of beer, lager, cider (even if you usually drink pints, calculate in half pints) ☐

  glasses of wine, sherry, vermouth ☐

  single measures of spirits (e.g. gin, vodka, rum, brandy, whisky)? ☐

Total ☐

Once the patient has completed the questionnaire, all you have to do is a quick calculation:

- Add up the number of units of alcohol on each drinking day.
- Multiply this number by the number of drinking days a week to discover the patient's total weekly consumption.

The amount of alcohol consumed should be recorded in the usual way, into the practice notes, or summary card.

One unit equals

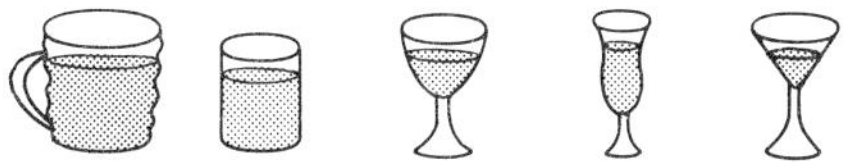

1/2 pint of ordinary beer, ordinary lager, or ordinary cider *OR* a single measure of spirits (whisky, gin, bacardi, vodka, etc.) *OR* a standard glass of wine *OR* a small glass of sherry *OR* a measure of vermouth or aperitif

Extra strong beers can have up to three times as much alcohol as ordinary beers.

Box 11.4: Converting your details

Low alcohol: Low-alcohol beers, lagers, ciders, and wines vary enormously in alcohol content. Some wines are as much as half the strength of ordinary table wine whilst the beers, lagers, and ciders listed are one-third of ordinary strength, but all can be as low as 0.05%—virtually alcohol free. All figures are approximate.

	Units	Percent alcohol content by volume (%ABV)
Low alcohol lager, beers and cider		0.5–1.2
Half pint	$\frac{1}{3}$	
1 pint	$\frac{2}{3}$	
1 can	$\frac{1}{2}$	
Beers, lager and cider		3.0–4.0
Ordinary strength		
Half pint	1	
1 pint	2	
1 can	$1\frac{1}{2}$	
Strong Ale, lager (premium), cider		4.1–6.0
Half pint	$1\frac{1}{2}$	
1 pint	3	
1 can	$2\frac{1}{4}$	
Extra strong beer, lager and cider		8.0–10
Half pint	$2\frac{1}{2}$	
1 pint	5	
1 can	4	
Table wine		11
1 standard glass	1	
1 standard bottle (75 cl)	8	
1 litre bottle	11	
Sherry and fortified wines		16
1 standard small measure	1	
1 bottle	13	
Spirits		40
1 standard single measure in England and Wales	1	
1 standard measure in N. Ireland and Scotland	$1\frac{1}{2}$	
1 bottle	30	

Note: 1 can = 16 fl. oz = 440 ml = $\frac{3}{4}$ pint.

Box 11.5: Patients who may be at risk from alcohol abuse

Select patients with any of the following characteristics:

- raised blood pressure;
- recurrent injuries or accidents;
- non-specific gastrointestinal complaints;
- marital or family problems;
- record of absenteeism;
- history of anxiety/depression;
- high-risk occupations (e.g. publicans, seamen, journalists).

Box 11.6: Selecting your patients who should cut down

Compare your patient's weekly consumption with the guidelines:

- **Lower risk**: Men 0–21/women 0–14 units a week. These totals can be recommended as reasonable limits for most adults (although they are too high for some see below), as long as the drinking is spread through the week, with at least two or three alcohol-free days. Encourage patients not to exceed these moderate levels for the sake of health and safety.
- **Raised risk—health warning**: Men 22–35/women 15–21 units a week. Try to keep patients in this category under fairly careful review as their drinking is approaching risky levels. You may want to point this out to them. Stress that drinking bouts increase the chances of accidents and injury.
- **Higher risk—advise to cut down**: Men 36 plus/women 22 plus units a week. We recommend that all patients drinking at this level should be advised to follow the programme to cut down. Damage to health is likely on this amount of alcohol, although the patient may not be aware of it yet. Drinking may also be affecting his or her work and personal life.
- **Lower for some**: much lower or zero limits are advisable for some: pregnant women, people being treated for high blood pressure, people who find it very difficult to control their drinking, people who are susceptible to alcohol because of extreme youth or old age, medication, ill-health.

Start by explaining the harm that can arise from too much drinking. Some of the problems include:

- raised blood pressure;
- headaches;
- stomach upsets;
- anxiety and depression;
- sexual difficulties;
- overweight;
- sleep problems;
- poor concentration—poor work performance;
- accidental injuries;
- liver disease;
- hangovers;
- cancers;
- irritability;
- financial worries.

Point out the positive reasons for drinking less:

- less risk of accidents, high blood pressure, or liver disease;
- the possibility of losing weight;
- improved concentration and a clear head;
- fewer hangovers, headaches, and stomach upsets;
- sounder sleep and less tiredness generally;
- more energy and time for new activities;
- fewer arguments and rows with friends and family;
- more pleasure out of sex;
- new sense of being in control of life and feeling fitter;
- if trying for a baby, improved chance of success for both men and women;
- extra cash.

If the patient is pregnant remind her that cutting down to one or two units a week, preferably giving up alcohol, will benefit the baby.

Use the drinking population chart (Fig. 11.1) to show the patient if their alcohol consumption is above average. Useful tips to give the patient planning to cut down are shown in Box 11.7.

Agreeing an action plan

A patient's ultimate target should be to keep within the weekly limits: 14 units of alcohol for women; 21 for men. Ten ways to cut down are shown in Box 11.8. Some people will want or need to abstain altogether. It is important that the patient agrees that the target is realistic, and for someone drinking very heavily a higher interim target might be set with a longer-term aim to cut down further. If a patient shows signs of dependence (e.g. withdrawal

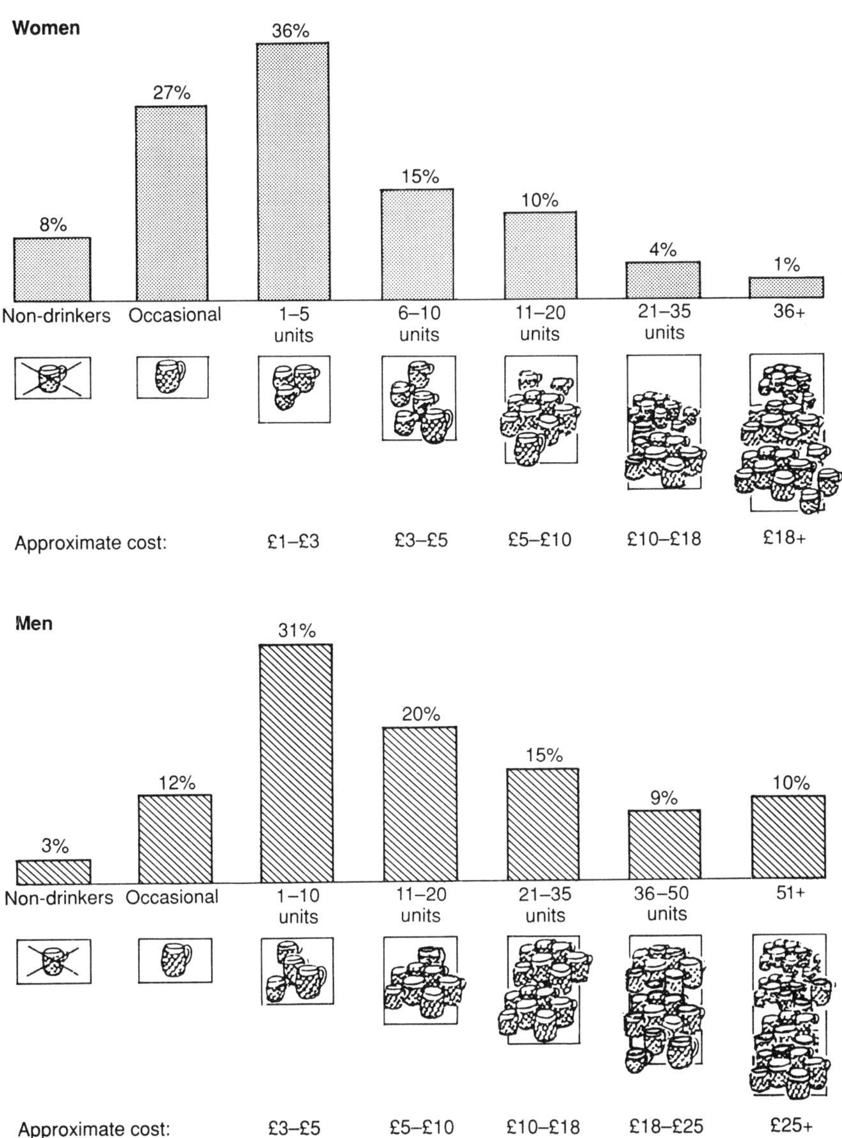

Fig. 11.1 Drinking population chart.

Box 11.7: Getting ready to cut down

The following eight points are useful tips for the patient in planning to cut down:

1. Choose a date in the next few days to cut down on drinking. Try to pick a day when you'll be under less stress.
2. Decide what weekly limit you're going to aim for. You may decide to cut down gradually over a few weeks. Eventually you may even decide to stop drinking altogether.
3. Plan to do things other than drinking: going to a film, playing sports or exercising, starting an evening class or doing some DIY at home. It is up to you. The important point is to find activities you enjoy which do not involve alcohol.
4. Use your drinking diary to find which times of day, where, and with whom you drink more than usual. You may sometimes drink to change your mood, for example when feeling tired, stressed, or anxious. You need to be prepared for these 'risk' situations and to plan your life differently at these times.
5. Try to get someone else to cut down on drinking with you. You could be a great help to each other.
6. Tell people you are cutting down and tell them when. They could be helpful too.
7. If you drink at home, stock up on plenty of alternatives to alcoholic drinks—such as alcohol-free beers and wines and other soft drinks. If you drink in pubs, find a low-alcohol or non-alcoholic drink that you enjoy.
8. Keep thinking about the positive reasons for drinking less and the benefits. If you really make up your mind, you will succeed.

symptoms, early morning drinking) he or she may need extra help and support in cutting down and may need to aim for abstinance rather than moderate drinking.

Encourage the patient to keep a regular drinking diary (Fig. 11.2) as a way of measuring progress and sticking to new limits. Stress the need to fill it in accurately.

If there is time, go through the last seven days' drinking together working backwards from today, noting down each day's drinking in units of alcohol and working out the weekly total. This will help make sure the patient understands how to use the diary and give them a baseline from which to assess progress.

Box 11.8: Ten ways to cut down

The following ten points are useful for the patient in helping to cut down.

1. **Keeping a drinking diary**. This helps you to control your drinking and stick within your target. You will be able to see which times and situations lead you to drink more—so if need be you can make changes to avoid them.
2. **Stick to your limit**. Work out a reasonable weekly limit for yourself, based on the drinking target—then stick to it. Set a limit for particular occasions too, like parties or the pub.
3. **Watch it at home**. Most drinks people pour at home are much more generous than pub measures, especially at parties. Take care not to go over your limit. Try to avoid heading straight for a drink when you get home: look for other ways to relax.
4. **It's OK to say no**. Don't be pressured into drinking by people who say 'Go on, have another one' or 'A little drink won't hurt you'. There's nothing wrong with choosing soft drinks or drinking less than other people.
5. **Avoid rounds**. Round buying often means you drink more than you want. Say you'd rather get your own, or, when it's your round, choose an alcohol-free drink for yourself.
6. **Occupy yourself**. Find something else to do whilst you drink—for example, playing darts, dominoes, pool, listening to music, chatting, eating (beware of salted snacks that make you thirsty). Any of these will distract you from the glass and help you to drink more slowly.
7. **Find alternatives**. Avoid drinking as a habit, because you're bored, feeling tense, or have nothing else to do. Look for other ways to relax or feel better.
8. **Have days off**. Keep at least two or three alcohol-free days a week. (This does not mean you can drink more on the other days: it's best to avoid binges.)
9. **Pace your drinks**. Sip slowly, and choose smaller drinks–a half instead of a pint. Try spacing out alcoholic drinks with soft drinks, or take lower-strength or alcohol-free drinks.
10. **Reward yourself**. Chart your progress. When you deserve it, give yourself a pat on the back. Cutting down on drinking requires willpower and self-control—you can be rightly proud of yourself for succeeding. Buy yourself a treat, using the money you save by drinking less. But be consistent: only reward yourself when you succeed with one of the targets you have set in advance.

Day	When	Where	What	Who with	Units
Total for the week					

Fig. 11.2 Your drinking diary for a week.

Follow-up action

Your patient's motivation will be strengthened if you can make clear that you will be following his or her progress in some way. If possible, arrange a follow-up appointment in two to four weeks' time. Ask them to bring the drink diary to this appointment, and to keep a note of anything they want to ask at that time. Should you not wish to offer another appointment, at lest make it clear that the patient will be asked about his or her drinking at the next consultation.

It is useful to put a reminder in the patient's notes to check his or her drinking in the future. Record the date when they stated the programme, the average weekly alcohol consumption at that time, and the target for cutting down.

Patients who find it too hard to cut down

On follow-up, some people may report that they have discovered that it is very difficult to reduce their drinking. It may be that they are physically dependent on alcohol, or more likely that they are used to drinking to cope with certain situations and have not yet found alternative ways of coping. Such patients may find it helpful to go for further advice to a specialist agency. If they are indeed physically dependent then a referral for detoxification may be indicated.

Further information on managing the problem or dependent drinker is given in the DRAMS pack and the Royal College of General Practitioners' publication, *Alcohol and drugs.*

References

Anderson, P. (1989). Self-administered questionnaires for diagnosis of alcohol abuse. *Diagnosis of alcohol abuse*, (ed. R. R. Watson). CRC Press. Boca Raton, Florida.

Anderson, P. and Scott, E. The effect of general practitioner advice to heavy drinking men. *British Journal of Addiction.* (In Press.)

Anderson, P., Cremona, A., Paton, A., Turner, C., and Wallace, P. (1991) The risk of alcohol. Submitted for publication.

Scott, E. and Anderson, P. (1990). Randomised controlled trial of general practitioners intervention in women with excessive alcohol assumption. *Drug and Alcohol Review*, **10**, 313–2.

Wallace, P., Cutler, S., and Haines, A. (1988). Randomised controlled trial of general practitioner intervention in patients with excessive alcohol consumption. *British Medical Journal*, **297**, 663-8.

Further reading

Alcohol and health: a handbook for nurses (1989). Medical Council on Alcoholism, London.

Hazardous drinking: a handbook for general practitioners (1987). Medical Council for Alcoholism, London.

Alcohol problems: practical guides for general practice (1988). Oxford University Press.

Alcohol—a balanced view (1986). Royal College of General Practitioners, London.

Alcohol and drugs (1991). Royal College of General Practitioners, London.

Management of drinking problems (1991). WHO Regional Publications, European series, No. 32. WHO Regional Office for Europe, Copenhagen.

Cut down on your drinking pack (1991). Health Education Authority, London.

For patients

The following are useful self-help books for patients with more extensive problems:

DRAMS pack (1989). Scottish Health Education Group, Edinburgh.

Miller, W. and Munoz, R. (1982). *How to control your drinking.* Sheldon Press, London.

Robertson, I. and Heather, N. (1986). *Let's drink to your health: a self-help guide to sensible drinking.* British Psychological Society. (Available from the British Psychological Society, The Distribution Centre, Blackhorse Road, Letchworth, Herts SG6 1HN)

Further information

Local services providing advice/information and treatment for people with alcohol problems varies. For information on what is available in your district contact your local alcohol treatment agency or look in the telephone directory under alcohol advice services.

12 Stress

Peter Anderson

Definitions

It is not easy to define stress. The word is used loosely; stress is used by different people to mean different things. The *Oxford English Dictionary* states that the word came into the English language from the old French word 'destresse', which meant to be placed under narrowness or oppression. In its Middle English form, the word was distress; over the centuries the word lost its 'di' giving us two words, distress and stress. These two words have come to have rather different meanings, the first indicating something unpleasant, the second something ambivalent.

The definition of stress adopted in this chapter is that of an external demand made upon the adaptive capacities of the mind and body. If these capacities handle the demand and enjoy the stimulation involved, then stress is welcome and helpful. If the capacities cannot handle the demand, then stress is unwelcome and unhelpful.

This definition means three things:

1. It makes clear not only that stress can be both positive and negative, but since there is a very wide range of things that can make demands upon the body and mind, there is a very wide range of things that can cause stress (stressors).
2. It suggests that it is not always events that determine whether individuals are stressed or not, but also their reactions to them.
3. Stress is a demand made upon the body's capacities. It is the nature and extent of capacities over which individuals have some control that influence their response to the demand. If the capacities are large enough, individuals may adapt, but if they are limited individuals are usually unable to respond.

To understand stress, it is necessary to look at external demands and how they can be influenced and at personal capacities and how they can be adapted. Just as demands can vary from situation to situation, so personal capacities can vary from individual to individual.

In practical terms what this means is that any person under stress must first look at the environment, to identify demands that are being made upon him or her and to see whether these demands can be altered or lessened in any way, and secondly, at himself or herself to see whether personal reactions to these demands can be similarly modified, by either increasing capacity or making use of what capacity is already available.

Size of the problem

Different methods are used to assess the number of people suffering from stress. However, there is no single reliable way of determining how common it is. Several related factors are used as an indication of the degree to which stress is present in the population.

Some people have conducted surveys on measures of stress such as unpleasant emotional strain in everyday life. Others have conducted surveys on stress-related issues, such as sleeping patterns and personality types.

In one British study (Ward and Payne 1982), respondents were asked if they had experienced 'unpleasant emotional strain yesterday'

All of the time	4%
Most of the time	5%
About half of the time	4%
Some of the time	7%
Just a little of the time	13%
Not at all	65%

Thirty five per cent of respondents experienced some stress on the day in question.

More than 5 million people consult their general practitioner (GP) each year because of mental ill-health (OPCS 1986). It is the second most common reason for consultation accounting for at least 15 per cent of all consultations. The two most common mental health problems presented by adults to their GPs are depression and anxiety. Women consult three times more often than men.

An indirect indicator of stress is the use of tranquillizers, which are usually prescribed as treatment for anxiety and insomnia. The main category of psychologically active medicines prescribed are benzodiazepines. In 1989, 22.1 million prescriptions for benzodiazepines were dispensed by community pharmacists.

Stress and health

A list of conditions attributed to stress is shown in Table 12.1.

Accidents

In several studies, it has been shown that accidents at home, on the roads, and at work are more likely to occur when individuals are under stress (Kalimo *et*

Table 12.1 Conditions associated with stress and anxiety

Social	Psychological	Physical
Overwork	Tiredness	Headaches
Use of drugs	Boredom	Backaches
alcohol	Depression	Poor sleep
tobacco	Irritability	Indigestion
illegal	Inability to concentrate	Chest pain
Accidents	Depression	Nausea/vomiting
Impulsive behaviour	Low self-esteem	Dizziness
Poor relationships	Apathy	Sweating
at home	Eating disorders	Trembling
at work	Tremors/stuttering	Palpitations
Poor work performance	Insomnia	Allergies
Assault	Obsessions/phobias	Aphthous ulcers
Marital and family break-downs	Nervous or mental break-downs	Arrhythmias
Social isolation	Suicide	Heart disease
	Self-poisoning	Strokes
	Sexual problems	Ulcers
	Sleep problems	Baldness
		Infections
		Colitis
		Constipation/diarrhoea
		Cystitis
		Dermatitis/eczema
		Indigestion
		Menstrual disorders
		Migraine
		Obesity
		Cancers

al. 1987; Cabinet Office 1987). This is probably because people are more easily distracted when abnormally anxious and do not take the same care with potentially dangerous tasks.

In a study of road users admitted to orthopaedic wards following road traffic accidents, it was found that drivers at fault had experienced significantly more stressful life events in the year preceding the accident than the group not at fault (Holt 1981).

Stress is also an important factor in industrial accidents. In another study (Levenson *et al.* 1983), 110 men and 54 women who had had industrial accidents were interviewed to assess what life events they had experienced in the year prior to the accident. For both sexes, increases in stressful life events had occurred prior to the accident.

Alcohol and tobacco use

In a study carried out in Stockholm to investigate the reasons for alcohol consumption among working people, a questionnaire was sent to key informants at work: company managers and chiefs, physicians, and the representatives of groups of workers in trade unions (Kuhlorn 1971) Work-related factors such as job dissatisfaction and time pressure together with marital problems featured as the most important reasons for drinking reported by the workers' representatives. The foremen regarded time pressure as the third reason in order of rank for alcohol consumption. The physicians placed work-related reasons such as time pressure and feelings of insecurity second in order of rank, following marital problems, which were regarded as the primary reason by all respondents.

Investigations in the police force in the UK indicate that high levels of work-related stress can facilitate the tendency of some individuals to drink heavily as a way of dealing with this kind of pressure (HEA 1988).

Smoking is more likely to persist under conditions of tension and anxiety. A relationship has been demonstrated between stress at work and smoking. A study of 35 000 nurses in the UK found that smoking was one of the most commonly identified ways of coping with stress (Hawkins *et al.* 1983). The decision to stop smoking in particular has been shown to be negatively related to various stresses. Inabilities to stop smoking in engineers and scientists have been associated with job stress and high levels of work load (Kalimo *et al.* 1987; Cabinet Office 1987).

Infections and immune system

Evidence suggests that stress impairs the workings of the immune system, which may lead to greater susceptibility to infections, including cold and influenza viruses. An interesting study of respiratory streptococcal infections illustrates the point. It was shown (Table 12.2) that streptococcal illness, streptococcal infections without illness, and non-streptococcal respiratory infections were about four times as likely to be preceded as followed by a stressful life event.

The results of recent studies have suggested that stress is significantly associated with subsequent infections, in particular those of the respiratory tract (Clover *et al.* 1989).

Cancers

Those who respond to stress by smoking or drinking more heavily will increase their risk of developing cancers of the oesophagus, larynx, and lung. It is also possible that some cancers might be produced as a result of a immune response within the body. Those who support this theory suggest

Table 12.2 Respiratory infections in families and their relation to acute stress. (From Meyer and Haggerty 1962)

	Episodes of acute stress (nos.)		Infections	
	2 weeks before	2 weeks after	Total number	Associated with stress
Streptococcal illness	17	3	56	30%
Streptococcal acquisition without illness	12	3	76	16%
Non-streptococcal respiratory infection	17	4	201	8%
Total	46	10	333	14%

that individuals who are particularly susceptible to stress are more likely to develop tumours produced by auto-immune responses (i.e. immunological reactions to our own body tissues). This is still an area for debate.

A major review covering 61 studies on the relationship between stress, cancer, and the immune system concluded that stress probably affects survival, or progress, of cancer more than it does initiation. However, new information on virus-induced cancer suggests that stress may increase cancer risk (Fox 1988).

Heart disease

Low socio-economic status, low social support, and employment characterized by high demands and low level of control over the job have been described as being associated with increased coronary risk (Krantz and Raisen 1988; Siltanen 1987; Williams 1987).

In the 1960s Friedman and Rosenman, found that coronary patients under study behaved similarly—they were aggressive, competitive, striving for achievement. These individuals were described as type A personalities, as opposed to more relaxed type B personalities (Rosenman *et al.* 1964; Burkeman 1988; Eaker 1989). The extent to which stress is a risk factor for coronary heart disease is not clear.

High blood pressure and strokes

High blood pressure is more common among people whose occupations expose them to frequent mental strains, excessive responsibilities, and conflicting situations.

The most extensively studied population in relation to the cardiovascular effects of psychosocial stress is air traffic controllers in the United States (Rose 1978). It was demonstrated that the incidence of raised blood pressure was three to four times greater in the controllers than in comparable workers in other occupations. A change from low to high workload was accompanied by modest statistically significant elevation in both systolic and diastolic pressures.

Assessment of stress and anxiety

Many people are good at hiding their stress from themselves as well as from everyone else. Even if friends and colleagues may be aware that an individual's judgement in important matters is suspect, it may be difficult to confirm. The individuals concerned may continue as they are, without acknowledging the strain that they are under, until they suffer psychologically or physically, or their inability to cope causes harm to others.

Organizations, and people within them, are often reluctant to take the problem of stress seriously. Many take an admission that an individual is under stress as a sign of weakness or inadequacy; individuals affected by stress may take the same view.

Individuals are all familiar with single or defined stressful events, such as moving house or changing jobs. In addition stress can accumulate gradually; i.e. from an increasingly demanding job, or from a mind or body that grows older, or because of progressive disease is less able to handle demands that at one time would not have been stressful.

Measurement of stress

There are a number of scales in existence to measure stress, in which respondents are asked whether they agree or disagree with certain statements about themselves. The responses are then given a numerical value and totalled (Powell and Enright 1990). The problem with such scales is that although the adverse consequences of too much stress are similar for most people, their reactions to them can be very different. For example, absenteeism from work increases generally when people are over-stressed. But some individuals may show a decrease in absenteeism, forcing themselves to go into work even when they are unwell, either through a need to prove themselves, or through a fear that decisions unfavourable to them will be taken if they are not around to protect their interests.

Scales of stress

Another problem with scales is that stress levels do not necessarily remain constant. An individual may score completely differently if tested at different times or in different situations. The circumstances in which stress occurs also vary from individual to individual.

Symptoms that can indicate stress are shown in Table 12.3 and scores for measuring the emotional, physical and work related effects of stress are shown in Appendix 12.1. These scales can be used to assess stress amongst patients and their results recorded in the notes.

Table 12.3 Symptoms that can indicate stress

Physical
- losing sleep
- headaches
- impotence
- muscle tension
- minor illnesses

Psychological/emotional/behavioural
- difficulty concentrating
- lack of self-worth
- more pessimistic and unhappy
- increased anxiety
- feeling tense and strained
- irritability
- indecision
- absenteeism

Social
- increased use of drugs, mainly alcohol and tobacco

Managing stress

Cognitive appraisals

Making the right cognitive appraisals helps individuals to alter thinking in more realistic and effective ways. And when individuals have looked at what it is in them that makes them an easy target for stress, decisions can be made on how they need to change, so that these decisions can be carried through successully. But there remains in many cases the problem of how to let thoughts adequately influence emotions.

Even in the most stressful of days there are many events that are not stressful at all. The actual bad moments may be relatively few in number. Often the problem is that these episodes dominate thinking and emotions throughout the day, to the extent that opportunities are missed to enjoy the much more frequent good moments. Good moments revive and relax individuals to make them better able to cope when the next episode of stress arrives.

Cognitive understanding of causation of stress is based on the underlying theory that an individual's mood and their behaviour are largely determined by the way she or he structures the world. One key component of increasing individual capacity is the ability to control thought processes.

Relaxation, in whatever form, will have a therapeutic effect. A non-competitive hobby, reading or listening to music, can produce relief. Some people, however, are unable to devote regular periods of time each day to such activities and for them a more formal, disciplined approach is necessary. This can include meditation or other forms of relaxation.

Meditation

Frequent and regular meditation, even if only for a few minutes a day, does four things that are helpful in a stress-reducing programme:

1. It trains the attention.
2. It increases control over thought processes.
3. It increases the ability to handle emotions.
4. It aids physical relaxation.

If properly used, meditation is one of the most helpful psychological techniques available in developing the resources needed to counter stress, anxiety, worries, and negative mental and emotional states. A meditation programme is shown in Appendix 12.2.

Human minds are easily distracted, and to introduce control, meditation selects a single object or experience and requires the meditator to stay calmly focused on it. As thoughts arise, they are not permitted to divert from the meditator's chosen object or experience. The meditator makes no attempt to push thoughts away or to stop them arising. The thoughts are simply denied attention. Whether the thoughts are good or bad, important or unimportant, they are allowed to pass in and out of the usual train of judgements and associations. If the mind does become distracted by a particular thought it is gently coaxed back to the point of focus, the moment the meditator realizes that this happened.

The point of focus on the object, or experience upon which the individual chooses to meditate, can be almost anything. Some traditions teach the use of what is called a mantra, a single word phrase which is repeated over and over again, to which full attention is given. Other use a mandala, a geometrical design upon which the meditator gazes with full attention.

One of the best techniques taught by other traditions is to use breathing. Attention is placed either upon the nostrils, where cool air can be felt entering on breathing in and warm air exhaling on breathing out, or concentration can be made upon the rise and fall of the abdomen. To help do this, it is often useful, particularly in the early stages, to count each breath going from one to ten and then back again to one, repeatedly.

People become less stressed by controlling their thoughts, instead of letting their thoughts always control them. Having become experienced with meditation, it is possible for individuals to deliberately let into their awareness the memory of some stressful experience they have had during the day. Usually the memory of this experience would bring an immediate emotional reaction. However, in the tranquility of meditation, the memory can come back without any emotional reaction. Instead of arousal, the individuals experience relaxation. It also allows individuals to be more honest about their emotions and to identify those occasions when in fact they have clung on to the emotion instead of relinquishing it. After some time, it is possible to realize that the emotion is very much less substantial than had been imagined. Also individuals begin to realise that the emotion itself is something for which they are ultimately responsible.

In the same way that meditation can deliberately switch awareness from breathing to emotions so it can also switch awareness from breathing to the body. This allows individuals to identify physical tensions that build up in their bodies during the day and then calmly let the tension go, through a system of exercises.

Other forms of relaxation

When relaxed, the mind and body are released from external stresses and become free of tension. Although this is a desirable aim, many people feel unable to relax or unwind and spend much of their waking lives feeling tensed and stressed. One of the major problems in getting people to relax is that so much of life is spent in activities that are perceived as desirable and individuals are seldom trained to 'switch off' and relax. As a consequence people often fail to spot evidence of tension and stresses in their bodies or overrule these feelings when they are perceived.

Other forms of relaxation are similar to meditation in that they lead to the same results through somewhat different means. Because muscles can be more easily trained to respond to conscious control the technique of progressive muscular relaxation can often be used. A programme for relaxation is shown in Appendix 12.3. A programme for coping with sleeping difficulties is shown in Appendix 12.4.

Physical activity

Stress often results when the body is geared for action but has no way of expressing it. Most normal stress is related to obvious danger and in the past the appropriate action was to face up to the danger or escape from it as quickly as possible. Both these activities were helped by the physical changes that take place under stress. Blood is transferred from parts of the body where it is not needed to the muscles and the heart where extra function is required. Physical activity is a way of responding to stress and allows the discharge of the energy the body is anticipating. Physical activity can be taken in many ways, including activities such as walking, jogging, dancing, or sport.

There is evidence that regular physical activity protects against stress-related conditions such as heart attacks. In general it is wise to embark upon programmes of steady exercise that involve regular activities rather than intermittent and strenuous sports such as weightlifting. It is also better to exercise as many muscles as possible, as in walking, running, and swimming. In addition to protecting against stress-related diseases regular activity helps to keep weight down (with its attendant benefits), and maintains joints and ligaments in good working order. People also feel better when fit and so self-confidence and self-esteem are improved.

Self-help materials for stress and anxiety

A wide range of self-help materials for stress and anxiety have been produced (Turvey 1985) and several of these have been evaluated in general practice (Kiley and McPherson 1986; Donnan *et al.* 1990). A package consisting of six separate leaflets containing information on the causes, consequences, and control of stress was studied in a randomized trial of patients presenting to their general practitioner with psychological problems which were potentially stress-related (Kiley and McPherson 1986). At three months' follow-up significant advantages were found for patients who received the package when compared with controls in both their level of symptoms and their rate of consulting for psychological problems.

In a second study a self-help package for anxiety was developed. The package consisted of a cassette audiotape and a printed booklet with four main sections (Donnan *et al.* 1990). Section one described what it feels like to be anxious, causes and consequences of anxiety, and an outline of ways to get over anxiety. Section two dealt with stopping anxiety developing. Section three summarized ways in which anxiety can be coped with better, including understanding the problem, dealing with the causes of anxiety where possible, using relaxation, coping with worry, planning better coping, having realistic expectations, letting other people help, and dealing with panic. Section four summarized the main points.

The package was evaluated using a randomized controlled trial. At three

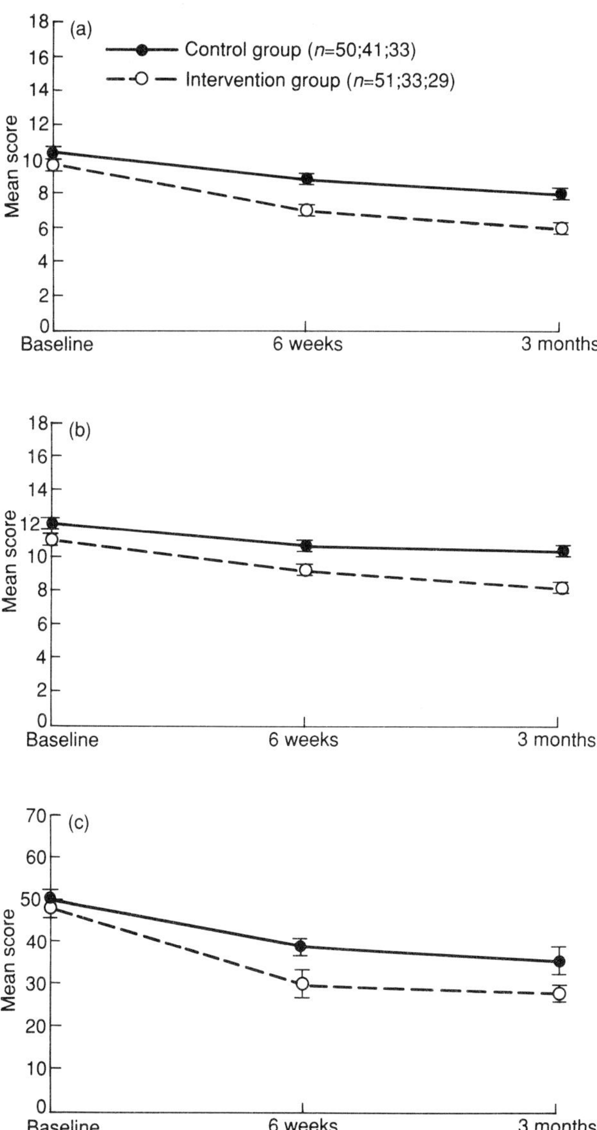

Fig. 12.1 Changes in mean outcome scores for the control and intervention groups on the three scales (n = number of patients in each group at each time point). (a) Mean Leeds self-assessment specific depression score. (b) Mean Leeds self-assessment specific anxiety score. (c) Mean general health questionnaire (Likert) score.

months follow-up the intervention was successful in terms of mean depression scores, mean anxiety scores and general health questionnaires which were lower for the intervention group than the controls (Fig. 12.1).

Use of benzodiazepines

The use of self-help packages is an alternative to prescribing benzodiazepines. Although the number of benzodiazepine prescriptions has been reduced, 22.1 million prescriptions were dispensed by community pharmacists in 1989.

Counselling in general practice has been shown to be effective in reducing anxiety and avoiding benzodiazepine prescribing. However, offering support in this instance is likely to be different from the support needed to help the dependent person come off benzodiazepines. An advice leaflet for coming off benzodiazepines is given as Appendix 12.5.

Following a study that took place in Oxford, it was concluded that there was little difference in outcome between samples of anxious patients in two group practices (Catalan *et al.* 1984). One sample received a benzodiazepine prescription, the other received counselling which was brief and unspecialized, consisting mainly of simple listening, explanation, advice, and reassurance. It appeared from this study that counselling did not make greater demands on the GP's time. The patients involved in counselling appeared to be more satisfied with their treatment than those receiving anxiolytic drugs and there was no increase in alcohol or tobacco consumption, nor a rise in the use of non-prescribed drugs.

Appendix 12.1: Emotional, physical, and work-related stress

Questionnaire 1: Am I suffering from the emotional effects of stress?

Tick the answer that most applies to you.

Often —More than once a week.
Sometimes—More than once a month.
Rarely —Less than once a month.

	Often	Some	Rare
Do I ever feel unable to cope?			
Do I find it difficult to relax?			
Do I ever feel anxious for no reason?			
Do I find it hard to show my true feelings?			
Am I finding it hard to make decisions?			
Am I often irritable for no real reason?			
Do I worry about the future?			
Do I feel isolated and misunderstood?			
Do I like myself?			
Am I finding it hard to concentrate?			
Am I worried about my health?			
Do I find that life has lost its sparkle?			

Scoring: Score one for every answer you have ticked in the 'often' box.

A score of 0–3 indicates slight stress.
A score of 4–6 indicates moderate stress.
A score of 7–11 indicates severe stress.
A score of 12 indicates very severe stress—you should seek medical help.

If you scored more than 3 then it indicates that your body is trying to adapt to stress. See these signs as a warning and take some action to reduce those things in your life which are causing your stress. Try this questionnaire again in a few months and see if there is any improvement.

Questionnaire 2: Am I suffering from the physical effects of stress?

Tick the answer that most applies to you.
Often —More than once a week.
Sometimes—More than once a month.
Rarely —Less than once a month.

	Often	Some	Rare
Do I ever have aching shoulders or neck muscles			
Do I have trouble sleeping?			
Do I have persistent indigestion?			
Am I feeling unusually tired?			
Is my blood pressure too high?			
Do I have unexplained dizzy spells?			
Do I smoke to calm my nerves?			
Do I eat erratically?			
Do I ever feel nauseous?			
Do I have a drink to unwind?			
Am I experiencing sexual difficulties?			
Do I have unexplained skin rashes?			

Scoring: Score one for every answer you have ticked in the 'often' box.

A score of 0–3 indicates slight stress.
A score of 4–6 indicates moderate stress.
A score of 7–11 indicates severe stress.
A score of 12 indicates very severe stress—you should seek medical help.

If you scored more than 3 then it indicates that your body is trying to adapt to stress. See these signs as a warning and take some action to reduce those things in life which are causing your stress. Try this questionnaire again in a few months and see if there is any improvement.

Questionnaire 3: Work performance

	Never	Rarely	Sometimes	Often	Always
I cannot get my work finished in time	1	2	3	4	5
I haven't the time to do things as I would like them to be done	1	2	3	4	5
I'm not clear exactly what my responsibilities are	1	2	3	4	5
I haven't enough to occupy my mind or my time	1	2	3	4	5
I don't get on with my boss	1	2	3	4	5
I lack confidence in dealing with people	1	2	3	4	5
I have unsettled conflicts with other staff	1	2	3	4	5
I get very little support from my colleagues or my superiors	1	2	3	4	5
I never know how I'm getting on in my job. There's no feedback	1	2	3	4	5
No one understands the needs of my department	1	2	3	4	5
Our targets/budgets are unrealistic and unworkable	1	2	3	4	5
I have to take work home to get it done	1	2	3	4	5
I have to work at weekends to get everything done	1	2	3	4	5
I can never take all my leave	1	2	3	4	5
I avoid any difficult situations	1	2	3	4	5
I feel frustrated	1	2	3	4	5
Total score =					

How do you score?

0–20 The stressors are about average for most people who enjoy their work but inevitably find things frustrating from time to time.

21–45 The stressors are such that you get tense and uptight from time to time and you will have to follow the relaxation techniques.

45+ The stressors are too high. Are you perhaps a type 'A' personality, a worrier or a perfectionist?

Appendix 12.2: Meditation programme

- Choose a time and a place where you are unlikely to be disturbed.
- Sit in an upright chair, or cross-legged on a firm cushion. Clasp your hands lightly in your lap. Keep your body upright. Don't allow the head or shoulders to sag, or your back to slump. Relax your muscles as much as possible.
- Close your eyes, and allow your attention to focus gently upon your breathing.
- Allow the sensation of breathing to occupy your full awareness. Whether you are focusing on your nostrils or your abdomen, keep the sensation of breathing as your point of focus. Do not shift from nostrils to abdomen or vice versa. Choose one point of focus and stick with it.
- Count silently 'one' on the first out-breath, 'two' on the second, 'three' on the third and so on until you get to ten. When you reach ten, count backwards on each out-breath until you get to one. Then back up again to ten and so on. If you loose track of your counting at any point, go back one and start again.
- When thoughts arise, neither follow them nor try to push them away. Do not label as 'good' or 'bad', whatever they contain. Simply keep your attention on your breathing. Allow thoughts to pass in and out of your mind without attending to them or hindering them.
- When the meditation session is over, rise slowly from your seat. Try to maintain something of the awareness experiences in meditation as you go about your day. Try to be aware of the sights and sounds around you in the same way you were aware of your breathing, without rushing to conceptualize about them or to pass judgements or to set off trains of association.

To begin with it does not really matter how long you sit in meditation. Regular daily practice at the same time each day is far more important than length of time. Usually it is helpful to start with five minutes a day and to gradually increase this over time to fifteen or twenty minutes a day.

It does not matter which time of day is used. Keeping to a set time is more important than when that time happens to be. Once the practice of meditation becomes established, in addition to the set times you can turn your attention to your breathing and feel yourself calming down whenever the day becomes stressful or whenever you want to do so. For, although meditation requires a set time and a set place and a set posture, if you are to train yourself properly in this technique, it does not have to be confined to those times. Meditation is simply the practice of awareness.

Appendix 12.3: Relaxation programme

When we are stressed, the muscles in our body become tense. When our muscles become tense, we may suffer from: headaches, stiff neck, painful shoulders, tight chest and difficulty breathing, trembling, racing heart, churning stomach, and tingling in our hands and face.

The most effective way of controlling body tension and stress is by relaxing. By relaxing, we don't mean sitting in front of the television or having a hobby. We mean developing a skill to reduce unnecessary physical tension. When our bodies are free of stress and tension, our minds tend to be relaxed.

However, the ability to relax is not something which always comes naturally. It is a skill which has to be learnt.

- In advance, try to decide when you are going to practice; in this way you can better develop a routine which you can stick to.
- Make sure that you choose somewhere quiet to practice, and make sure that no one will disturb you.
- Don't attempt to practice if you are hungry or have just eaten, or if the room is too hot or too cold.
- Start by lying down in a comfortable position;
- Adopt a 'passive' attitude; don't worry about whether you are relaxing or not.
- Try to breathe through your nose, using your stomach muscles. Try to breath slowly and regularly.

Longer programme

Use this programme first. When you have mastered it move on to the shorter programme.

First, tense your muscles as hard as you can. Really concentrate on the feelings of tension and strain. Hold this for a few seconds and relax. Notice the difference, think how your muscles feel when they are relaxed. Focus on the sensations in your muscles each time you tense and relax them. The relaxation exercise involves doing this for all parts of your body.

Feet:	Pull your toes back, tense your feet muscles. Relax and repeat.
Legs:	Straighten your legs, point your feet towards your face. Relax and repeat.
Abdomen:	Tense your stomach muscles by pulling them in. Relax and repeat.
Back:	Arch your back. Relax and repeat.

Shoulders: Shrug your shoulders as hard as you can, bringing them up and in. Press your head back. Relax and repeat.

Arms: Stretch out your arms and hands. Relax and repeat.

Face: Think about tensing your forehead and jaw. Lower your eyebrows and bite hard. Relax and repeat.

Whole body: Tense your entire body, hold for a few seconds. Repeat and relax.

Breathe slowly and regularly between tensing and relaxing each part of the body.

When you have completed the exercise, spend a few moments relaxing your mind. Close your eyes. Think about something restful. Breathe slowly through your nose. Continue for a minute or two, then open your eyes. Do not stand up straight away, and when you feel ready move slowly and stretch gently.

Shorter programme

When you are able to use the longer programme successfully, you can use the shorter programme by missing out the 'Tense' stage. You can progress through the routine by just relaxing the different muscle groups. When you can do this, you can use the programme at other times and in other places. For example, you might try it in a sitting position, rather than a lying position; or you might move from a quiet room in the house to a noisier room.

When you are able to achieve a relaxed state using the above two programmes, you can begin to practice applying these skills throughout the day.

Through the day remember to:

- drop your shoulders;
- relax the muscles in your body;
- check your breathing pattern;
- relax.

Appendix 12.4: Coping with sleeping difficulties

Sleeping difficulties are common. As many as one in five people complain of difficulty in falling asleep, of waking during the night, or early morning wakening. These experiences can be quite normal and only become a problem when you worry about them.

Some facts about sleep which are useful to know are:

1. There is no such thing as an ideal length of sleep: some people need ten hours and some need four.
2. As you grow older, you require less sleep.
3. Everyone has 'broken sleep' in that we all wake several times during the night, and simply go back to sleep.
4. There is no danger in losing a few nights of good sleep.
5. Sleep can be affected by many things; stress, mood, exercise, food, medicines, and alcohol. By altering your behaviour you can take control of your sleeping pattern without resorting to drugs.

Why avoid drugs?

Sleeping tablets are addictive. An occasional sleeping pill, might be useful in the short term. However, your body quickly comes to rely on them and very soon it is difficult to sleep without tablets. When you try to stop taking them, you can find that your sleep pattern is worse than ever and that you want to revert to taking the pills.

Helping to get to sleep

1. Relax: no-one has unbroken sleep and everyone has the odd period of poor sleep. If you don't worry you will sleep better.
2. Prepare yourself before going to bed. This should involve:
   - taking exercise during the day;
   - avoiding spicy or heavy food and caffeine (tea or coffee) in the few hours before you go to bed;
   - taking time to relax by having a warm bath, listening to restful music, reading a book, or completing a relaxation exercise;
   - making sure your bedroom is quiet;
   - emptying your bladder.
3. Go to bed when you are sleepy.
4. When you are in bed, relax and do not think about worrying issues. Use your relaxation programme.

Appendix 12.5: Coming off benzodiazepines

1. When you start to cut down, you may experience unpleasant symptoms. The common symptoms are, tremor and shaking, intense anxiety, panic attacks, dizziness and giddiness, feeling faint, an inability to get to sleep, and an inability to sleep throughout the night, an inability to concentrate, nausea, a metallic taste in the mouth, depression, headaches, clumsiness and poor coordination, sensitivity to light, noise and touch, tiredness and lethargy, a feeling of being outside your body, blurred vision, hot and cold feelings, and a burning on your face, aching muscles, an inability to speak normally, hallucinations, sweating and fits.
2. These symptoms can be minimized by reducing the dose slowly. The rate at which the dose is reduced will depend upon the size of dosage you have been taking. One easy rule is that the dose should be halved every two weeks until it can no longer be halved. Then the drug can be cut out altogether. The higher the dose you are taking the longer it will take to wean yourself off the pills completely. It can take many months.
3. Benzodiazepines cure nothing, but they do cover symptoms up. If you originally took your tablets for anxiety, then the chances are your original symptoms will be returned. Be prepared for this and look at the issues covered elsewhere in this book on how to cope with stress.
4. Before giving up you may or may not need to visit your doctor and seek help too.
5. Don't try to give up if you are going through a difficult time, wait until things are somewhat more settled before trying to give up.
6. Warn your family and friends that you are likely to be going through a difficult time. Tell them what to expect and explain that you will need extra support, sympathy, and patience. It is important to keep in touch and share your problems.

References

Burkeman, R. T. (1988). Obesity stress and smoking: their role as cardiovascular risk factors in women. *American Journal of Obstetrics and Gynaecology*, **158**, 1592–7.

Cabinet Office (1987). *Understanding stress*, part one. HMSO, London.

Catalan, J., Garth, D., Edmonds, G., and Ennis, J. (1984). The effects of non-prescribing in general practice: 1. Controlled evaluation of psychiatric and social outcome. *British Journal of Psychiatry*, **144**, 593–603.

Clover, R. D. *et al.* (1989). Family functioning and stress as predictors of influenza B infection. *Journal of Family Practice*, **28**, 535–9.

Donnan, P., Hutchinson, A., Paxton, R., *et al.* (1990). Self-help materials for anxiety: a randomized controlled trial in general practice. *British Journal of General Practice*, **40**, 498–501.

Eaker, E. D. (1989). Psychological factors in the epidemiology of coronary heart disease in women. *Psychiatric Clinics of North America*, **12**, 167–73.

Fox, B. H. (1988). Epidemiological aspects of stress, ageing, cancer and the immune system. *Annals of the New York Academy of Sciences*, **521**, 16–28.

Graham, N. M., *et al.* (1986). Stress and acute respiratory infection. *American Journal of Epidemiology*, **124**, 389–401.

Hawkins, E., *et al.* (1983). Smoking, stress and nurses. *Nursing Mirror*, October, 3.

Health Education Authority (1988). *Stress in the public sector.* Health Education Authority, London.

Holt, P. L. (1981). Stressful Life events preceding road traffic accidents. *Inquiry*, **13**, 111–15.

Kalimo, R., El-Batawi, M., and Cooper, C. L. (ed.) (1987). *Psychological factors at work.* World Health Organization, Geneva.

Kiley, B. C. and McPherson, I. G. (1986). Stress self-help packages in primary care: a controlled trial evaluations. *Journal of the Royal College of General Practitioners*, **36**, 307–9.

Krantz, D. S. and Raisen, S. E. (1988). Environmental stress, reactivity and ischaemic heart disease. *British Journal of Medical Psychology*, **61**. 3–16.

Kuhlorn, E. (1971) Alcohol and work. *Alkohol Praagen*, **65**, 222–30.

Levenson, H., *et al.* (1983). Recent life events and accidents; the role of sex differences. *Journal of Human Stress*, **9**, 4–11.

OPCS (1986). *Morbidity statistics from general practice 1981–1982. HMSO, London.*

Powell, T. J. and Enright, S. J. (1990). Anxiety and stress management. Routledge, London.

Rose, R. M. (1978). *Air traffic controller health change study.* United States National Technical Information Service.

Rosenman, R. H., *et al.* (1964). A predictive study of CHD. *Journal of the American Medical Association*, **189**, 15–22.

Siltanen, P. (1987). Stress, coronary disease and coronary death. *Annals of Clinical Research*, **19**, 96–103.

Turvey, A. (1985). Treatment manuals. In *New developments in clinical psychology*, (ed. F. N. Watts). British Psychological Society, London.

Warr, P. and Payne, R. (1982). Experience of strain and pleasure among British adults. *Social Science and Medicine*, **16**, 1691–7.

Williams, R. B. (1987). Psychological factors in coronary heart disease: epidemiologic evidence. *Circulation*, **76**, 1117–23.

13 Exercise

Archie Young

There is nothing new about the idea that ill-health may be prevented by regular physical exercise. What is new is the increasing body of evidence which confirms the salubrious effects of exercise or at least indicates that exercise has physiological effects which are potentially beneficial (Åstrand and Grimby 1986; Fentem *et al.* 1988; Bouchard *et al.* 1990).

Increasing awareness of the health benefits of regular exercise has led to a variety of campaigns intended to encourage the general public to adopt a more active lifestyle. Public reaction to these has been mixed. There are cynics who assume that if official bodies are advocating exercise, there must be a flaw. Their arguments are fuelled by newspaper stories of the more bizarre hazards of jogging, such as being struck by lightning or developing penile frostbite. A Member of Parliament has even gone so far as to recommend that tracksuits should carry a government health warning 'Danger—jogging can kill', seeming to imply that regular physical activity should be equated with cigarette smoking. In contrast, a growing number of people seem interested in the idea that exercise might not only promote good health but that it might also be fun to do. This response has been much more marked in the upper social classes, just as they have responded best to education about the health hazards of smoking.

People are now approaching their general practitioner with a request for advice on the relationship between exercise and health. In order to answer these questions effectively, the general practitioner must not only be up to date on the available scientific evidence but must also be aware of the prevailing popular beliefs or 'myths' about exercise. For example, a widely held, lay view is that exercise which causes breathlessness is intrinsically harmful!

General benefits of regular exercise

Regular exercise can increase endurance, strength, suppleness, and skill. This reduces the disturbance of the resting state which is required to perform everyday activities, thereby also reducing the subjective sense of effort. The nature of the training exercise determines the nature of the adaptations which occur.

Improved endurance

Aerobic (or oxygen-using) exercise is exercise conducted at a submaximal intensity for periods upwards of five minutes. Repeated bouts of such exercise constitute 'endurance training' and produce adaptations throughout the oxygen transport system. These are both central and peripheral adaptations. Physiologists delight in debating their relative importance.

Centrally there is little or no change in lung volumes (at least in the adult) but the heart gets both larger and stronger and ventricular emptying during exercise becomes more complete. Blood volume and total body haemoglobin both increase.

Peripherally, there is an increase in the ability of the working muscles to extract oxygen from their blood supply. Contributing factors include an increase in the oxidative enzyme content of the muscle fibres. The latter is reflected morphologically by an increase in the number, size, and complexity of muscle mitochondria. These changes are more pronounced in the muscles, and even in the individual muscle fibres, which were used most during the training exercise.

The same intensity of exercise will therefore require a smaller flow of blood through the working muscles and correspondingly less diversion of blood away from the splanchnic bed. There will be a smaller rise in peripheral resistance and a correspondingly smaller increment in arterial blood pressure.

Unless there has been an improvement in skill or exercise technique, a given intensity of aerobic exercise will require the same level of oxygen uptake post-training as it did pre-training. This level of oxygen uptake, however, will be achieved with a lower ventilation and a lower heart rate after training than before and the sensation of effort is less for a given work rate after training.

Increased strength

Appropriate training can increase the strength of a muscle. Strength training comprises a relatively small number of maximal or near-maximal muscle contractions. Except for the specialist athlete, it is probably of little importance whether these contractions are isometric or isotonic—that is whether the muscle's length is unchanged or whether the force is unchanged. There are two possible exceptions to this: (i) isometric contractions may sometimes be preferable in order to produce a training effect without irritating a painful joint or a soft-tissue injury; (ii) isometric contractions may sometimes be relatively contraindicated on account of their tendency to produce large elevations of blood pressure; this will be discussed in more detail later. What is important is that improvement in the performance of a strength-related task is very much greater if the task has been practised than after merely increasing the intrinsic strength of the muscles involved.

Increased suppleness and skill

Regular repetition of appropriate types of movement will also improve suppleness and neuromuscular coordination (skill). As with strength and endurance these benefits will be specific to the nature of the training exercise.

Benefits in old age

Regular exercise is no elixir of youth, but it can go a long way towards reducing the level of impairment which is all too readily accepted as being synonymous with old age. For example, loss of muscle strength (especially in the presence of joint disease) may mean that an elderly person is no longer able to use a bath unaided or is unable to avoid a fall if she stumbles on an uneven surface. Diminished aerobic fitness may mean that climbing the hill to the shops produces an unacceptable degree of tachycardia and tachypnoea. Appropriate physical training, however, can increase the elderly person's strength and/or aerobic exercise capacity at least as readily as in young people (Young 1992; Greig and Young 1992).

Hypothermia is an important cause of mortality and morbidity among elderly people. The elevation of the metabolic rate which persists after the cessation of exercise may well reduce the risk of hypothermia.

Regular physical exercise is not merely beneficial for elderly people. It may be critical for some in determining whether or not they retain their independence (Bassey 1978; Young 1992; Greig and Young 1992).

Benefits of exercise when chronic disease is present

Physical training reverses the effects of inacivity due to the typical, modern lifestyle. In patients with chronic disease, however, the effects of immobility can be even more severe; patients may have been immobilized by doctors or by their own perception and (mis)understanding of their symptoms. For example, if a patient's disease is such that symptoms occur during exercise (e.g. dyspnoea in chronic bronchitis) he will tend to avoid physical activity (Fig. 13.1). The loss of physical fitness which results from his inactivity results in the occurrence of symptoms at progressively lower levels of exercise, even though the fundamental physical impairment due to the disease remains unchanged (i.e. he gets breathless more easily, despite an unchanged peak expiratory flow rate). This 'vicious circle' can spiral through so many revolutions that a patient with only moderate disease becomes severely disabled by his low exercise tolerance. Such a 'vicious circle' applies in many different situations, but can be seen very clearly when dealing with patients with chronic airways obstruction, angina, or peripheral arterial insufficiency. As doctors, we are insufficiently alert to the extent to which the physiological effects of immobility contribute to our patients' symptoms and disabilities.

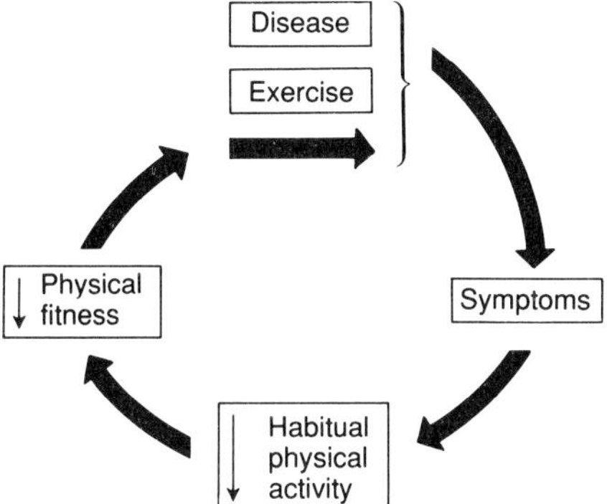

Fig. 13.1 'Vicious circle' that may ensnare patients with exercise-related symptoms, with the result that their symptoms are provoked by progressively lower levels of exercise. (From Young 1981)

Psychological benefits of exercise

Physical training has been incorporated into therapeutic programmes for patients with recognized psychiatric disorders. For example, it has been argued that 'any rational, safe, and effective treatment regime for depression should include a prescription for vigorous exercise'. Physical recreation is also rewarding for many mentally handicapped people. Nevertheless, I believe that the major psychiatric role for regular exercise (preferably as recreational sport) is not so much in the treatment of established psychopathology, but rather in the prevention of anxiety, depression, boredom, and self-deprecation in the 'normal' population. In addition, exercise with a team or club ensures important opportunities for informal psychological support.

This is one of the most difficult areas in which to conduct satisfactory scientific studies to validate the claims made for exercise. Nevertheless, there is reasonably good evidence that regular aerobic exercise may result in improved sleep, reduced anxiety, and reduced depression. These changes are seen at their best in patients participating in a therapeutic exercise programme and whose anxiety and depression are related to the physical impairment resulting from their medical condition. For example, following a myocardial infarction one of the principal justifications for the inclusion of physical exercise in a rehabilitation programme is the improvement which it produces in confidence and self-esteem (Hackett and Cassem 1973).

Specific preventive benefits of regular exercise

Ischaemic heart disease

Primary prevention This is probably the area in which regular exercise has its most important role in the primary prevention of disease. It has been reviewed recently by Froelicher (1990) and new evidence continues to accumulate (e.g. Morris *et al.* 1990). The evidence will never be absolutely complete; a controlled trial of exercise in the prevention of coronary heart disease would mean totally dictating the lifestyle of several thousand people for at least five to ten years.

There is a great weight of evidence in favour of a protective effect of exercise against coronary heart disease and I consider the case proven 'beyond reasonable doubt'. Those who disagree usually do so with one of four arguments. I shall comment on each of these in turn.

The classical studies of Morris and his colleagues into the exercise habits and ischaemic heart disease experience of transport workers and civil servants and of Paffenbarger and his colleagues with San Francisco dockworkers showed that men whose daily life involved vigorous physical activity were less likely to suffer myocardial infarctions and were still less likely to die from them. This kind of study can easily be criticized on the grounds that men with undiagnosed, premorbid ischaemic heart disease might have tended to select lighter jobs and leisure activities. Morris has now gone a long way towards discrediting this counter-argument with his demonstrations that up to nine years after the survey, those men who had reported participation in vigorous exercise continue to have a more favourable coronary heart disease experience (Morris *et al.* 1980, 1990).

Secondly, it is sometimes claimed that inactivity, if statistically isolated from all other influences, seems to be a relatively weak 'risk factor' for coronary heart disease. In fact, the studies of Paffenbarger and of Morris indicate that inadequate exercise has a similar valency to other major risk factors. Moreover, this kind of analysis, by definition, only evaluates a hypothetical, intrinsic effect of exercise itself. It does not take into account the fact that physical training influences several other risk factors, changing all of them in a 'protective' direction. Thus, physical training may lower the circulating concentrations of 'pathogenic', very-low-density-lipoprotein triglyceride and low-density-lipoprotein cholesterol, may increase 'protective' high-density-lipoprotein cholesterol, increases the fibrinolytic reponse to vascular occlusion, may lower blood pressure slightly, decreases ventricular ectopic activity, reduces the myocardial oxygen consumption required to perform a standard amount of external physical work, helps to regulate weight, improves glucose tolerance, and perhaps even discourages the wish to smoke.

Thirdly, it is sometimes argued that there is no point in encouraging a patient to exercise if the 'risk factor' dice are already loaded against him. Why bother persuading him to start swimming if he is not going to stop smoking? Once again, Morris has the answer—'in virtually every situation we have studied, favourable or unfavourable, men engaged in vigorous sports or recreations . . . had about half the coronary attack rates of their fellows.' This is also borne out by Paffenbarger's work.

The fourth counterargument offered can be summarized as 'It's too late to start, the damage has already been done'. Yet Morris' latest work shows that men already aged 55–64 at the start of the study obtained the expected cardioprotective benefit over the ensuing nine years of follow-up. Moreover, Paffenbarger has data confirming that it is current activity that matters, not lifelong activity (Paffenbarger, personal communication).

Secondary and tertiary prevention Physical training allows a given level of external work to be performed at a lower heart rate and a lower arterial blood pressure than before training. Physical training therefore reduces the oxygen requirements of the myocardium and thus allows a greater level of external work to be performed before the onset of angina.

The importance of physical training for the post-coronary patient is more controversial (Shephard 1981). Nevertheless, authoritative opinion is in favour of including exercise training as part of a multifacetted programme of coronary rehabilitation (Froelicher 1990). Angina of effort can be improved or prevented, exercise tolerance increased, the psychological sequelae of a heart attack (principally anxiety and depression) reduced, and a sense of well-being produced. Perhaps there may also be a modest reduction in mortality for patients participating in a post-coronary exercise programme (Froelicher 1990). Supervised exercise in a group may be particularly useful since it allows the patient convenient and informal access to the 'health professional' running the class. Many patients also derive considerable psychological support from membership of a group of people who have been confronted with similar problems.

Supervised, group rehabilitation involving regular attendance at a hospital gymnasium would usually be prohibitively expensive. It is probably also unnecessary for all but a few patients. An arrangement which is more widely applicable is that the group should train at a local sports centre, under the guidance of a general practitioner. It is surely better for someone's self-image that they should attend a public sports centre rather than a hospital. There might also be a better chance that they will continue to be physically active. In one such scheme, the 'graduates' from the class meet during a public session immediately before the class. This maintains their contact with the class and also encourages those who have just joined the class.

Peripheral arterial insufficiency

Patients with longstanding, intermittent claudication can increase their claudication distance by following a programme of regular walking exercise (e.g. Larsen and Lassen 1966). The beneficial effect of regular exercise in a patient with stable peripheral arterial insufficiency is not due to an increase in calf muscle blood-flow during submaximal work. It is due to the trained muscle's greater ability to extract oxygen from its blood supply—the same adaptation that endurance training produces in normal muscle.

Hypertension

Mild or moderate hypertension is ameliorated by regular aerobic exercise (Hagberg 1990). It is not known whether the sequelae of hypertension are more or less frequent when the pressure has been reduced by exercise than when it has been reduced by drugs. At least regular exercise does not cause impotence, diabetes, and cold extremities.

There are two points to remember about drugs, hypertension, and exercise: (i) normal doses of sympatholytic drugs do not prevent the sudden and large increase in blood pressure which can be produced by isometric exercise (see 'Hazards'); (ii) the heart rate cannot be used as a guide to the intensity of exercise in a patient being treated with a beta-blocker.

Airways obstruction

Once again, the emphasis is on tertiary prevention. The beneficial effects of regular physical exercise for patients with chronic airways obstruction are well described in the literature (e.g. Grimby and Skoogh 1980; Editorial 1980) and their value in tertiary prevention was underlined by a report from the Royal College of Physicians of London (1981). There is also a useful pamphlet for patients (McGavin *et al.* 1979).

The benefits are probably due to a combination of reversal of the effects of inactivity, reduction of the fatiguability of the respiratory muscles themselves, and an increased psychological tolerance of breathlessness. Grimby calls the last of these mechanisms 'physical habituation' rather than 'physical training'. Its importance must not be underestimated; even if it is 'only a placebo effect' to the physiologist, it still represents a major reduction in the patient's disability.

It is also important that the child with asthma should be able to enjoy the general benefits of improved physical fitness and be relieved of the stigma of seeming less able than his peers. In addition, there is some evidence, albeit rather weak, which suggests that children with asthma may also derive other, more specifically therapeutic, benefits from regular swimming training, e.g. a lower bronchodilator consumption and a lower frequency of exacerbations.

In order that the child with asthma may participate to the full in physical recreation, it may well be necessary for his doctor to give appropriate advice on the choice of sporting activity and the optimal use of drugs in order to prevent exercise-induced asthma. In most patients, exercise-induced bronchoconstriction can be prevented by the inhalation of salmeterol or disodium cromoglycate during the half-hour preceding exercise. Games with an intermittent pattern of running (e.g. football, hockey, etc.) are usually rather less asthmogenic than continuous running and, since exercise-induced bronchoconstriction is precipitated by heat loss through the bronchial mucosa, the warm humid atmosphere in an indoor swimming pool greatly reduces the likelihood of provoking an attack. Many young people with asthma have been able to achieve international success as swimmers. Exercise is also of great benefit to adults with asthma (Young 1981), even to those who are steroid dependent (Afzelius-Frisk *et al.* 1971).

Obesity

Regular exercise assists weight regulation but is of little help to weight loss by those who are severely obese (e.g. Garrow 1986; Bray 1990; Garfinkel and Coscina 1990).

Weight reduction programmes which include both dietary restriction and regular physical activity may be more acceptable (and therefore more effective) than those which concentrate on dietary restriction alone, since the severity of dietary restriction can be less. It is not only during exercise itself that calorie expenditure is elevated, the metabolic rate may be elevated for several hours after the cessation of exercise. Some believe that this becomes particularly important if the exercise occurs regularly and frequently. Body fat can be significantly reduced by an exercise programme comprising 40 minutes vigorous walking four times a week.

Diabetes mellitus

Immobility results in impairment of glucose tolerance. Physical training restores this to normal. Further training enhances peripheral insulin sensitivity, i.e. it has an 'insulin-sparing' effect. Practical experience is that the control of maturity-onset diabetes may be improved by regular physical activity. This is due to a training-induced increase in insulin sensitivity (Holloszy *et al.* 1986).

Exercise also has beneficial metabolic effects for the patient whose diabetes is well controlled with insulin; it should be an integral part of his management (e.g. Felig and Koivisto 1979). Exercise may, however, aggravate the hyperglycaemia and hyperketonaemia of the insulin-requiring diabetic whose condition is poorly controlled (e.g. Berger *et al.* 1977).

Patients requiring insulin for the control of their diabetes also meet some practical problems when exercising. In particular, exercise may greatly increase the absorption of insulin from subcutaneous injection sites in the exercising limb. Absorption from other subcutaneous sites is unchanged or even reduced and the use of a nonexercised site is recommended to reduce exercise-induced hypoglycaemia. The adjustment of insulin dose and carbohydrate intake for periods of exercise lasting over an hour should be made with specialist guidance.

Osteoporosis

Disuse results in a loss of strength in bone. When a limb is immobilized in plaster, it takes only a few months for localized osteoporosis to become apparent.

Regular physical training can be used to increase the strength of the skeleton (Smith and Raab 1986; Tipton and Vailas 1990). For example, calcium loss from the os calcis was prevented during the third Skylab mission by requiring the astronauts to perform an exercise which entailed the repeated application of force to the bone by strong, resisted contractions of the triceps surae (Whittle 1979). Similarly, considering a problem more closely related to everyday life, it seems that regular exercise reduces the loss of calcium from bone in postmenopausal women. The sites of enhanced calcium deposition are specific to the pattern of physical stress applied to the skeleton. It is not only a bone's mineral content that increases in response to a repeated physical stress. Its internal architecture also changes, further increasing its mechanical strength to withstand that specific stress.

Arthritis

Of all the significantly disabled people aged 15–65 years, nearly one-third owe their disability to some form of arthritis. It is unlikely that exercise can make much contribution to primary prevention in this area. There may, however, be some scope for secondary and tertiary prevention. For example, it is widely accepted that the worst degrees of spinal deformity in ankylosing spondylitis can be prevented by adherence to a regular programme of stretching and mobilizing exercises, ideally in combination with regular swimming.

Muscular weakness is a common clinical problem in the presence of joint disease. It may contribute to further joint injury. Isometric exercises, as prescribed by physiotherapists, can increase muscle strength, even in the presence of rheumatoid arthritis. The restoration of strength is likely to be faster and more complete if joint pathology (swelling and/or pain, in particular) is well controlled (Young and Stokes 1986). Isometric exercise is used in the expectation that dynamic exercise would aggravate joint pain and inflammation. Nevertheless, a group of patients with ankylosing spondylitis reported diminished pain and joint stiffness after a four-week course of intensive, dynamic, physical training, namely 3–5 hours daily of swimming, gymnastics, hiking, cross-country skiing, horseback riding, and spinal exercises. It seems likely that we could safely encourage patients with arthritis to participate more fully in recreational sport, provided they choose activities which will not jar painful joints. This would help to prevent a 'disabled' self-image and to restore muscle strength and aerobic fitness without damaging the joint.

Back pain

A large, prospective study of Los Angeles firemen showed that back 'injuries' (undefined) were more common the lower the level of physical 'fitness' (defined as a composite score including measures of aerobic performance, lifting strength and spinal mobility) (Cady *et al.* 1979). It is not clear, however, which component of fitness contributes most to the prevention of back injury. Nor is it known to what extent these findings may be extrapolated to people in sedentary occupations. There is very little published evidence of the efficacy of exercise in preventing or treating lower back pain. For specific therapy, there is evidence that treatment with isometric flexion exercises is better than treatment with either flexion/mobilization or extensor-strengthening exercises but it is not known if it is any better than no treatment at all. In a more general approach, measures to encourage physical activity may be associated with a better overall outcome (Nachemson 1990). Nevertheless, as Nachemson (1976) has pointed out, 'It is known that . . . when lifting and carrying heavy objects . . . contraction of abdominal and costal muscles will help to relieve some of the load of the lumbar spine'. Moreover, the quadriceps take more weight in 'correct' lifting than in 'incorrect' lifting. Therefore, the logical inference is that strengthening abdominal, costal, and quadriceps muscles will relieve the load on the lumbar spine and so contribute to the prevention or amelioration of low back pain. Accordingly, many rheumatologists advise patients with recurring low back pain to take up regular swimming.

Hazards of exercise

Sudden death

How big a risk? In addition to extolling the benefits to be derived from recreational exercise, it is important that this chapter should also examine the possibility that vigorous exercise may be associated with an increased risk of unwanted side effects, the most important of which is sudden death. Much of the evidence has been reviewed by Siscovick (1990).

Deaths associated with vigorous exercise are most commonly due to ischaemic heart disease, subarachnoid haemorrhage, or congenital abnormalities of the coronary and great vessels. Deaths from subarachnoid haemorrhage may be related to sudden bursts of heavy work, which probably produce a sharp rise in blood pressure. There is little that could be done to avoid these deaths.

Of greater importance for the general population is whether vigorous exercise can cause sudden death from ischaemic heart disease. Sudden death during sport tends to attract the attention of the press but is, in fact, very rare. Vigorous exercise carries only a very small absolute risk; a study from Rhode Island gives a figure of approximately one death per 7600 middle-aged joggers, half of whom had a pre-mortem diagnosis of ischaemic heart disease. Nevertheless, this was still seven times the death rate during sedentary activities. A Seattle study supports these figures (Table 13.1) but also puts the increased risk during exercise into perspective. Among habitually vigorous men, the overall risk of sudden cardiac death, i.e. both during and not during vigorous activity, was only 40 per cent of that among sedentary men. Moreover, the risk of vigorous physical activity (whether sporting or non-sporting) was about 10 times as great among habitually inactive men as among the habitually most active group. Thus, vigorous physical activity carries a transiently increased risk of sudden cardiac death which is greatest in those who are habitually least active and which is outweighed in those who are habitually most active by a deceased overall risk.

The estimates of the importance of viral myocarditis as a cause of exercise-associated sudden death vary considerably from report to report. There is good experimental evidence from work with animals to suggest that it would

Table 13.1 The relative risk of sudden cardiac death during vigorous physical activity by middle-aged men with no clinically recognized coronary heart disease

Source	Habitual frequency of high-intensity exercise	Overall (24 hour) incidence of sudden cardiac death (per 10^8 person-hours)	Relative risk during high-intensity exercise	
			Mean	95% confidence limits
Thompson *et al.* (1982)	High or very high	Not known	3.5	2–13
Siscovick *et al.* (1984)	Very high	5	5	2–14
	High	6	13	5–32
	Low	14	56	23–131
	Nil	18	—	—

be unwise to exercise while suffering a viral infection since this may activate an otherwise transient, subclinical myocarditis.

The place of exercise electrocardiography in prevention There is a widespread belief in both medical and lay circles that the safety of exercise can be increased by undergoing an electrocardiographically monitored exercise test before starting training. This is fallacious and the reasons have been very clearly set out by Epstein (1979): 'In patients who, by history, have a high retest likelihood of coronary artery disease: 1. a positive electrocardiographic exercise-test result is of marginal diagnostic importance because it only slightly increases an already high likelihood of coronary disease; 2. a negative result in these same patients is valueless clinically because of the very high percentage of patients with false-negative results.' Moreover, with subjects who have a low pre-test likelihood of coronary artery disease, a positive response is often false positive and a negative response does not rule out the presence of significant disease. To have a chance of postponing the death of one asymptomatic middle-aged jogger per year, one would have to perform at least 15 000 tests, 10 per cent of which would be abnormal. This implies at least 1000 false positives, an epidemic of iatrogenic cardiac handicap.

The public must be enabled to recognize for themselves whether they are 'at risk' from coronary heart disease, when to seek medical advice, and that a normal exercise ECG is not a licence to ignore the advice to start gently and build up gradually.

The place of public education in prevention The average, untrained individual is indeed subject to a temporary increase in risk when he takes vigorous exercise. It seems likely, however, that the level of risk can be greatly reduced by starting the training programme with a very light level of exercise and making only small and gradual increments. Thus, as fitness improves, the relative strain imposed on the body increases very slowly indeed; any suggestion of untoward symptoms can be noted and acted upon. It is important that the lay public is educated to recognize the signs of an ischaemic myocardium being exercised too close to its limits. This is an area where family practitioners and national bodies responsible for health education must combine forces. It is essential that the jogger knows to seek medical advice if he experiences syncope or chest pain during exercise, or palpitations associated with shortness of breath or chest pain during exercise or shortly afterwards.

The Royal College of Physicians of London and the British Cardiac Society (1976) stated that 'Few need to consult their doctors before making a graded increase in their physical activity'. It is important that those who do need to consult their doctor can be identified or, more properly, can identify themselves (see Fig. 13.2). They can then be given any particular advice which is necessary for them to exercise safely, effectively, and enjoyably.

CONSULT YOUR DOCTOR IF:

1. You are under regular or recent medical treatment

OR 2. You've ever had high blood pressure, heart disease, chest pain, or an irregular heartbeat

OR 3. A close blood relative has had a stroke or a heart attack under the age of 50

OR 4. You're more than three stones overweight

OR 5. You smoke

OR 6. You're worried whether exercise may affect any other aspect of your health

Fig. 13.2 Suggested guidelines to permit self-identification of those who should consult their doctors before making a graded increase in their physical activity.

Popular marathons and mass runs

General practitioners may well be asked to advise local clubs or charities on the organization of a mass run, or to provide medical cover. This is not a responsibility to be taken lightly. Some of the essentials, notably hypovolaemia, hyperthermia and hypothermia, have been reviewed elsewhere (Young 1987). Detailed guidance or advice to participants and on the number, preparation, and disposition of staff are also available (Tunstall-Pedoe 1984).

Hazards of isometric exercise

Isometric exercise involves muscle contraction without movement, e.g. holding a heavy weight or trying to push an immovable object. It is often advised that isometric exercise should be avoided by those who might be thought to be susceptible to ischaemic heart disease or cerebrovascular problems. This is because isometric work produces a very large rise in blood pressure.

It must be remembered, however, that the concomitant increase in heart rate is very small and, as a result, the increase in the rate × pressure product is actually smaller during high-intensity isometric work with small muscle groups than with submaximal dynamic work with large muscle groups even though the increase in arterial blood pressure may be greater with isometric exercise. Since myocardial oxygen consumption depends more on the rate × pressure product than on the blood pressure alone, it is probably increased less by the isometric exercise.

It may be that isometric work is less dangerous for the myocardium than is usually stated. Nevertheless, isometric exercise can still produce two potential hazards: (i) when performing isometric exercise it is no longer appropriate to use the heart rate as a guide to myocardial oxygen consumption although this can be done during dynamic work; (ii) myocardial oxygen consumption can be pushed very high indeed by a combination of isometric exercise with a small muscle group (e.g. hand grip) and dynamic work performed with large muscle groups (e.g. brisk walking). Classically, this arises when the middle-aged, obese, hypertensive, aggressive business-executive tries to hurry through an airport terminal carrying his suitcase.

Muscular hazards

Stiffness Muscle stiffness 24–48 hours after unaccustomed exercise is the result of damage to muscle cells (rhabdomyolysis). The important practical points are that muscle stiffness can be minimized by making only a slow and gradual increase in the level of exercise and being particularly cautious about the amount of exercise involving eccentric muscle contractions (i.e. contractions in which the muscle is being lengthened despite being active . . . e.g. the quadriceps during the landing phase of squat-jumps). Training which includes small numbers of eccentric contractions affords protection against future damage of this sort.

Severe rhabdomyolysis is extremely rare, but potentially catastrophic. The resulting myoglobinuria may cause tubular necrosis and renal failure. It is seen most commonly in military recruits made to perform many repetitions of an unaccustomed exercise which puts a very high stress on a limited number of muscles. The patient with the so-called 'squat-jump syndrome' complains of painful 'stiff' muscles, is unwell and passes 'Coca-Cola'-coloured urine or may already be anuric. He should be managed by measures to encourage a large output of alkaline urine while arrangements are being made for his immediate transfer to hospital.

Cramp Additional salt is probably completely irrelevant for the prophylaxis of the vast majority of muscle cramps experienced in temperate climates. From a practical point of view, the important things to know are that cramp can usually be relieved by stretching the muscle and that regular training seems to reduce the incidence of muscle cramps.

Over-use syndromes

Excessively severe training, or an attempt to increase the training load too rapidly, can result in one or more of a variety of 'over-use' syndromes. Since running is the commonest form of exercise for 'keep-fit' athletes, the lower limbs are commonly affected (Fig. 13.3).

In the acute phase, these injuries should be treated by cessation of exercise and the prescription of a non-steroidal anti-inflammatory agent for a few days. Exercise should then be resumed at a much lower intensity and should be

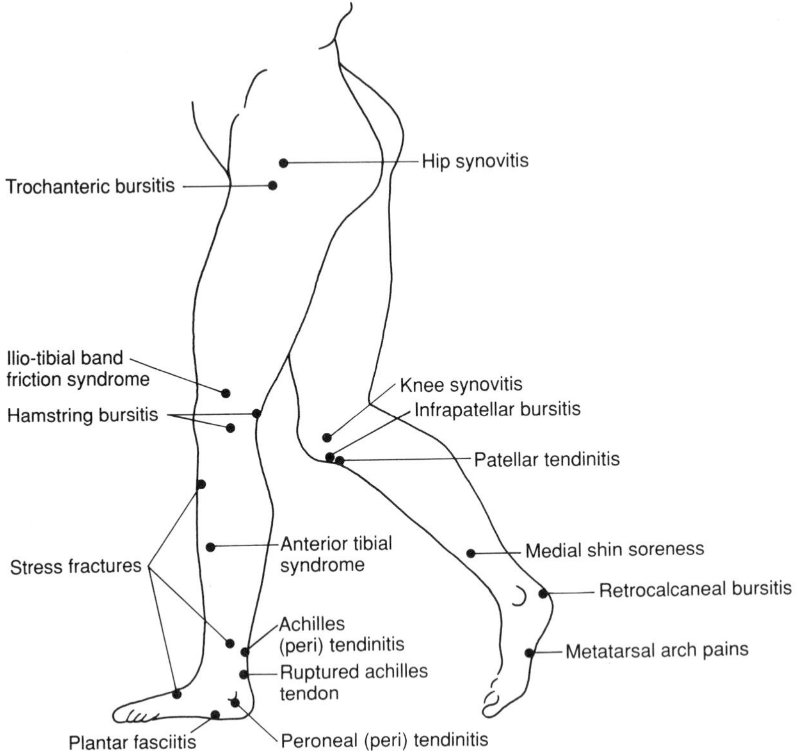

Fig. 13.3 Common sites of overuse injuries in joggers and runners.

increased more slowly than before. Very occasionally, additional treatment may be advised using, for example, ultrasound or the local infiltration of steroids.

Once established, over-use injuries can prove difficult to shake off and it is therefore preferable that they should be prevented. As already indicated, the most important factor in preventing over-use injuries is careful control of the rate of increase of the training load. Recurrent problems are an indication for a close examination of the athlete's technique.

Head injuries

The medical profession has an important role in the prevention of sports injuries due directly or indirectly to features of the equipment or the tactics (legal or illegal) used. The association between injuries sustained in rugby football and illegal practices is a good example (Davies and Gibson 1978).

How long will it be until the medical officers of all contact sports insist on players waiting four weeks after loss of consciousness before participating again—the rule which applies in amateur boxing? Such a step is overdue since it has been clearly shown that psychological function is impaired for two to three weeks after injuries producing even just a brief period of unconsciousness and that the effects of repeated injuries of this sort are cumulative.

The exercise prescription

Form of exercise

Most of the health benefits of exercise result from activities which train the oxygen transport system. These are activities which use large muscle groups and whose performance requires a large proportion of the maximal capacity of the oxygen transport system. This means brisk walking (progressing gradually to jogging and perhaps even to running), cycling, swimming, or a programme of 'physical jerks' such as the Canadian Air Force 5BX and XBX systems.

Although they too can bring their problems, the repetitive movements of swimming and cycling cause much less trouble than running since the body weight is supported in both these activities. This is particularly important for people who are overweight or who have a history of back or other joint symptoms. Even for those who are not overweight, weight-brearing exercises should mean the use of shoes with a thick, shock-absorbing cushion under the heel. Similarly, joggers should avoid hard surfaces and, wherever possible, run on grass.

Duration of exercise

The first few minutes of exercise are performed with the aid of the body's oxygen stores and by using the body's ability to exercise for a brief period without the use of oxygen (anaerobic exercise). As a result, the oxygen transport system can only be trained by exercise which lasts for more than just a few minutes—a minimum of ten minutes is preferable.

Intensity and frequency of exercise

A significant, aerobic-training effect can be achieved without exercising at the limit of capacity. Excessive zeal results in injuries which, although trivial in themselves, effectively prevent any further training for a week or two.

An endurance training programme should be started at an extremely low level of exercise—so low that the former athlete may be embarrassed by it. Over the age of 30 years, the first two to three weeks of a jogging programme should consist of nothing more strenuous than walking. Ten to twenty minutes of vigorous walking three times a week will produce a significant training effect. Subsequently, brief periods of jogging can be introduced at intervals during the walk. The relative properties of jogging and walking can then be gradually reversed.

Once a basic level of aerobic fitness has been achieved, the training exercise should be performed at some 60–70 per cent of the maximal oxygen uptake. During submaximal dynamic exercise, the heart rate (expressed as a function of the individual's resting and maximum heart rates) is a reliable indicator of the percentage of his maximal oxygen uptakes being utilized. The heart rate can therefore be used to check whether the training exercise is sufficiently, but not excessively, vigorous. This sort of approach is commonly advocated in North America. I feel, however, that it is unduly introspective and, moreover, there is evidence that it is not very reliable in practice. A perfectly adequate guideline for most people is that the exerise should be sufficiently strenuous for them to be aware that they are breathing more heavily. In the words of the Royal College of Physicians of London and the British Cardiac Society (1976) 'Getting breathless some time every day is a good habit'. The level of exercise which will be achieved by someone following this guideline will cross the training threshold sufficiently often for the desired effect to be achieved.

In order to ensure that the training intensity is not excessive, it is necessary also to have a guide to the upper limit of exercise intensity which should be attempted by someone unaccustomed to exercise. The Sports Council's guideline—'Run at talking pace'—is very satisfactory. Ventilation during exercise should not be so great as to prevent the athlete from carrying on a conversation while continuing to exercise.

The frequency with which endurance training should be performed depends to a large extent on the intensity and duration of each exercise session. For someone pacing himself as described above, the exercise should be continued for at least 10 minutes at a time, three times a week. Some may choose to fit their training exercise into the normal working day. Certainly it should not be too difficult to include a minimum of ten minutes of deliberately brisk walking on three occasions in the working week. This is not to say that important benefits might not be gained from less exercise, although they might be hard to confirm statistically. It is important that we are not too dogmatic in our assertion of the minimum amount of training exercise; some exercise is better than no exercise.

If the chief purpose of the exercise programme is to aid weight-loss, the intensity of activity may remain fairly low if the individual bouts are longer and more frequent. This might mean walking for an hour a day, five days a week.

'Behaviour modification' and the prescription of therapeutic exercise

The prescription of graded physical training is an important part of tertiary prevention for many patients. Motivation, however, can be a problem. It is often difficult to persuade a patient that he really will benefit from physical training. Even when the patient agrees that training would be worthwhile, sustained compliance can be very difficult. Sometimes, an increased level of 'exercise behaviour' can be encouraged by applying the elementary principles of 'behaviour modification' (Series and Lincoln 1978). An exercise 'class', whether in general practice or in hospital, can be planned in such a way that attention, rest and feedback of progress may all be used as 'reinforcers' to increase the frequency of 'exercise behaviour'. The length and severity of the work periods in each patient's exercise prescription can be adjusted so that, for example, a rest period is a 'reward' for the successful completion of a period of exercise, rather than being the consequence of an inability to continue the exercise. Oldridge and Jones (1986) discuss their attempts to improve compliance by such devices as spouse participation, written agreements, and giving the patient control of the exercise prescription.

In a person who has been inactive for a long time, the physiological effects of even a small amount of training may be dramatic. Fitness testing can therefore be used to provide the patient with evidence of progress and so reinforce his exercise behaviour. To do this successfully the trainer must know the adaptive capacities of the attributes to be tested and the variability to be expected in repeated tests. If tests are too frequent, small improvements will be concealed by random variation and exercise behaviour will be discouraged.

The general practitioner's contribution

If the medical profession accepts that there are significant health benefits to be gained from regular physical exercise, then it is morally bound to try and influence popular behaviour accordingly. 'Preventive medicine' becomes virtually synonymous with 'health education'. The public must be informed about the various ways in which regular exercise promotes health and the wide range of people (including patients) who can benefit.

The major public-health argument for advocating an increase in physical activity is the contribution that this would make to reversing the epidemic of coronary heart disease. Indeed, it can be argued that lack of vigorous exercise is so widespread that, in terms of population attributable risk, is much the most important influence on mortality from coronary heart disease. Statistically, it may account for 30–40 per cent of all deaths from coronary heart disease (Centers for Disease Control 1990). I doubt, however, whether the individual layman would see this as a sufficiently powerful argument for him to change his own, personal level of physical inactivity. A guarantee of immunity would be ideal, but a mere reduction in the likelihood of suffering a catastrophe at some unspecified time in the future is not an effective 'sales pitch'. Whilst we must inform the public about the role of exercise in the prevention of coronary heart disease, our emphasis should be on the early, positive benefits which can be guaranteed to come from physical training.

Having convinced people that they, personally, stand to gain something from regular exercise, the next responsibility is to ensure that they may exercise safely and that they continue to exercise. Newcomers to exercise must be educated in the recognition of untoward, exercise-related symptoms and the action to take if they occur. They must be taught how to avoid the troublesome aches and pains that may result from misguided enthusiasm or inappropriate equipment. Doctors must be able to give the right advice and guidance.

Acknowledgements

I am very grateful to several friends who were kind enough to criticize an early draft of this chapter, namely Professor J. N. Morris and, in general practice, Drs K. and E. M. Armstrong and Drs J. and A. N. Noble.

References

Afzelius-Frisk, I., Grimby, G., and Lindholm, N. (1977). Physical training in patients with asthma. *Le Poumon et le Coeur*, **33**, 33–7.

Åstrand, P.-O. and Grimby, G. (ed.) (1986). Physical activity in health and disease *Acta Medica Scandinavica* **Suppl. 711.**

Bassey, E. J. (1978). Age, inactivity and some physiological responses to exercise. *Gerontology*, **24**, 66–77.

Berger, M., Berchtold, P., Cüppers, H. J., Drost, H., Kley, H. K., Müller, W. A., *et al.* (1977). Metabolic and hormonal effects of muscular exercise in juvenile type diabetics. *Diabetologia*, **13**, 355–65.

Bouchard, C., Shephard, R. J., Stephens, T., Sutton, J. R., and McPherson, B. D. (eds.) (1990). *Exercise, fitnes, and health: a consensus of current knowledge*. Human Kinetics, Champaign, Illinois.

Bray, G. A. (1990). Exercise and obesity. In *Exercise, fitness, and health: a consensus of current knowledge*, (ed. C. Bouchad *et al.*), pp. 497–510. Human Kinetics, Champaign, Illinois.

Cady, L. D., Bischoff, D. P., O'Connell, E. R., Thomas, P. C., and Allan, J. H. (1979). Strength and fitness and subsequent back injuries in firefighters. *Journal of Occupational Medicine*, **21**, 269-72.

Centers for Disease Control (1990). Coronary heart disease attributable to a sedentary lifestyle-selected States, 1988. *Morbidity and Mortality Weekly Report*, **39**, 541–4.

Davies, J. E. and Gibson, T. (1978). Injuries in Rugby Union football. *British Medical Journal*, **2**, 1759–61.

Editorial (1980). Exercise and the breathless bronchitic. *The Lancet*, **ii**, 514–15.

Epstein, S. E. (1979). Limitations of electrocardiographic exercise testing., *New England Journal of Medicine*, **301**, 264–5.

Felig, P. and Koivisto, V. (1979). The metabolic response to exercise: implications for diabetes. In *Therapeutics through exercise* (ed. D. T. Lowenthal, K. Bharadwaja, and W. O. Oaks), pp. 3–20. Grune and Stratton, New York.

Fentem, P. H., Bassey, E. J., and Turnbull, N. B. (1988). *The new case for exercise*. The Health Education Authority and The Sports Council, London.

Froelicher, V. F. (1990). Exercise, fitness, and coronary heart disease. In *Exercise, fitness, and health: a consensus of current knowledge* (ed. C. Bouchard *et al.*) pp. 429–50. Human Kinetics, Champaign, Illinois.

Garrow, J. S. (1986). Effect of exercise on obesity. I *Physical activity in health and disease*, (ed. P.-O. Åstrand and G. Grimby) *Acta Medica Scandinavica* **Suppl. 711**, 67–73.

Garfinkel, P. E. and Coscina, D. V. (1990). Discussion: exercise and obesity. In *Exercise, fitness, and health: a consensus of current knowledge*, (ed. C. Bouchard *et al.*), pp. 511–15. Human Kinetics, Champaign, Illinois.

Greig, C. A. and Young, A. (1992). Aerobic exercise. In *Oxford textbook of geriatric medicine* (ed. J. G. Evans and T. F. Williams). Oxford University Press.

Grimby, G. and Skoogh, B.-E. (1980). Rehabilitation of the respiratory patient. In *Recent advances in respiratory medicine*, No. 2 (ed. D. A. Flenley), pp. 225–35. Churchill Livingstone, Edinburgh.

Hackett, T. P. and Cassem, N. H. (1973). Psychological adaptation to convalescence in myocardial infarction patients. In *Airlie conference on exercise testing and training of coronary patients*, (ed. J. Naughton and K. K. Hellerstein), pp. 253–62. Academic Press, New York.

Hagberg, J. M. (1990). Exercise, fitness, and hypertension. In *Exercise, fitness, and health: a consensus of current knowledge*, (ed. C. Bouchard *et al.*), pp. 455–66. Human Kinetics, Champaign, Illinois.

Holloszy, J. O., Schultz, J., Kusnierkiewicz, J., Hagberg, J. M., and Ehsani, A. A. (1986). Effects of exercise on glucose tolerance and insulin resistance. In *Physical activity in health and disease*, (ed. P.-O. Åstrand and G. Grimby), *Acta Medica Scandinavica* **Suppl. 711**, 55–65.

Larsen, O. A. and Lassen, N. A. (1966). Effect of daily muscular exercise in patients with intermittent claudication. *The Lancet*, **ii**, 1093-6.

McGavin, C. R., McHardy, G. J. R., and Lloyd, E. L. (1979). *Exercise can help your breathlessness.* Chest, Heart, and Stroke Association, London.

Morris, J. N., Everitt, M. G., Pollard, R., Chave, S. P. W., and Semmence, A. M. (1980). Vigorous exercise in leisure time: protection against coronary heart disease. *The Lancet*, **ii**, 1207–10.

Morris, J. N., Clayton, D. G., Everitt, M. G., Semmence, A. M., and Burgess, E. H. (1990). Exercise in leisure time: coronary attack and death rates. *British Heart Journal*, **63**, 325–34.

Nachemson, A. (1976). A critical look at conservative treatment for low back pain. In *The lumbar spine and back pain*, (ed. M. Jayson), pp. 355–65. Pitman Medical, London.

Nachemson, A. L. (1990). Exercise, fitness, and back pain. In *Exercise, fitness, and health: a consensus of current knowledge*, (ed. C. Bouchard *et al.*), pp. 533–40. Human Kinetics, Champaign, Illinois.

Oldridge, N. B. and Jones, N. L. (1986). Preventive use of exercise rehabilitation after myocardial infarction. In *Physical activity in health and disease*, (ed. P.-O. Åstrand and G. Grimby), *Acta Medica Scandinavica*, **Suppl. 711**, 123–9.

Royal College of Physicians of London and British Cardiac Society (1976). Prevention of coronary heart disease. *Journal of the Royal College of Physicians of London*, **10**, 213–375.

Royal College of Physicians of London (1981). Disabling chest disease: prevention and care. *Journal of the Royal College of Physicians of London*, **15**, 69–87.

Series, C. and Lincoln, N. (1978). Behaviour modification in physical rehabilitation. *British Journal of Occupational Therapy*, **41**, 222–4.

Shephard, R. J. (1981). *Ischaemic heart disease and exercise.* Croom Helm, London.

Siscovick, D. S., Weiss, N. S., Fletcher, R. H., and Lasky, T. (1984). The incidence of primary cardiac arrest during vigorous exercise. *New England Journal of Medicine*, **311**, 874–7.

Siscovick, D. S. (1990). Risks of exercising: sudden cardiac death and injuries. In *Exercise, fitness, and health: a consensus of current knowledge*, (ed. C. Bouchard *et al.*), pp. 707–13. Human Kinetics, Champaign, Illinois.

Smith, E. L. and Raab, D. M. (1986). Osteoporosis and physical activity. In *Physical activity in health and disease*, (ed. P.-O. Åstrand and G. Grimby), *Acta Medica Scandinavica* **Suppl. 711**, 149–56.

Thompson, P. D., Funk, E. J., Carleton, R. A., and Sturner, W. Q. (1982). Incidence of death during jogging in Rhode Island from 1975 to 1980. *Journal of the American Medical Association*, **247**, 2535–8.

Tipton, C. M. and Vailas, A. C. (1990). Bone and connective tissue adaptations to physical activity. In *Exercise, fitness, and health: a consensus of current knowledge*, (ed. C. Bouchard *et al.*), pp. 331–44. Human Kinetics, Champaign, Illinois.

Tunstall-Pedoe, D. (ed.) (1984). Popular marathons, half marathons and other long distance runs: recommendations for medical support. *British Medical Journal*, **288**, 1355–9.

Whittle, M. W. (1979). Exercise and the astronauts. *Medisport*, **1**(6), 12–15.

Young, A. (1981). But of course, exercise wouldn't help me!—physical conditioning for patients and normal subjects. In *Good health—is there a choice?*, (ed. P. H. Fentem), pp. 37–50. Macmillan, London.

Young, A. (1987). Sports medicine. In *Oxford textbook of medicine*, (ed. D. J. Weatherall, J. G. G. Ledingham, and D. A. Warrell), pp. 26.1–26.8. Oxford University Press.

Young, A. (1992). Strength and power. In *Oxford textbook of geriatric medicine*, ed. J. G. Evans and T. F. Williams). Oxford University Press.

Young, A. and Stokes, M. (1986). Reflex inhibition of muscle activity and the morphological consequences of inactivity. In *Biochemistry of exercise*, 6th edn, (ed. B. Saltin), pp. 531–44. Human Kinetics, Champaign, Illinois.

14 High blood pressure

Theo Schofield

Introduction

Measuring patients' blood pressures is probably the oldest established and most commonly performed item of preventive care in general practice. Patients receiving treatment for high blood pressure are the largest single group receiving continued care. The epidemiology of high blood pressure and its status as a major predictor of arterial disease is well established. The costs and benefits of treatment at different levels of blood pressure and indifferent age-groups have been studied in major clinical trials. There is therefore both a good reason and a good opportunity to create a clear policy for the measurement and management of high blood pressure in general practice.

Definition and prevalence of high blood pressure

Within the population there is a distribution of levels of blood pressure; some individuals will have pressures that are higher than others. In middle-aged men and women, about 20 per cent will have diastolic pressures in excess of 95 mmHg and between 4 and 5 per cent will have pressures of 110 mmHg or over. Studies based on single readings may exaggerate the prevalence, which also increases with age.

Apart from the very small number of hypertensive patients who have renal disease or endocrine disorders, these individuals do not have a 'disease' (Fig. 14.1a) but are just at the upper end of the distribution curve. The dividing lines between hypertension that justifies treatment, moderate hypertension that requires risk factor management and follow-up, but not necessarily treatment, and the rest of the population are arbitrary (Fig. 14.1b). They are based on the balance between the risks of that level of blood pressure and the risks and benefits of intervention and treatment. The evidence of these will now be considered.

The risks of high blood pressure

The major risks associated with high blood pressure are heart attack, stroke and heart failure. High blood pressure may also contribute to the development of peripheral artery disease, cerebral arteriosclerosis, and renal failure.

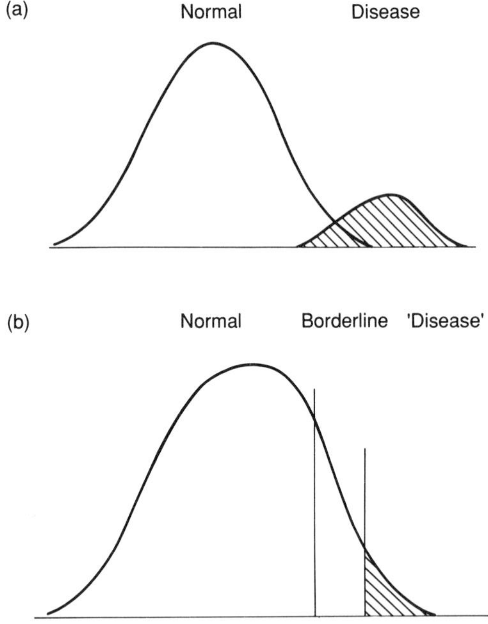

Fig. 14.1 Population blood pressure distribution.

Malignant hypertension is an uncommon, but severe, consequence of high blood pressure. The scale of the risks associated with high blood pressure can be expressed in a number of ways.

Relative risk

Life insurance statistics and early epidemiological studies expressed the risks of a person with high blood pressure as a multiple of the risks of the population as a whole. Mortality increases steadily with increase in blood pressure. A man with a blood pressure of 140/90 has a mortality about 50 per cent above average, of 145/95 a mortality about double average, and of 160/100 about three times average mortality. These relative risks are more marked in younger patients (Fig. 14.2a). But blood pressure measurements for insurance purposes and in observational studies have often been recorded once only and these readings may substantially underestimate the association between level of blood pressure and mortality because of 'regression dilution bias'. This is because there are random fluctuations of blood pressure over time, and repeated measurement results in readings at the top and bottom of the distribution moving towards the average value. The effect of this bias is to systematically underestimate the strength of the real association (MacMahon *et al.* 1990).

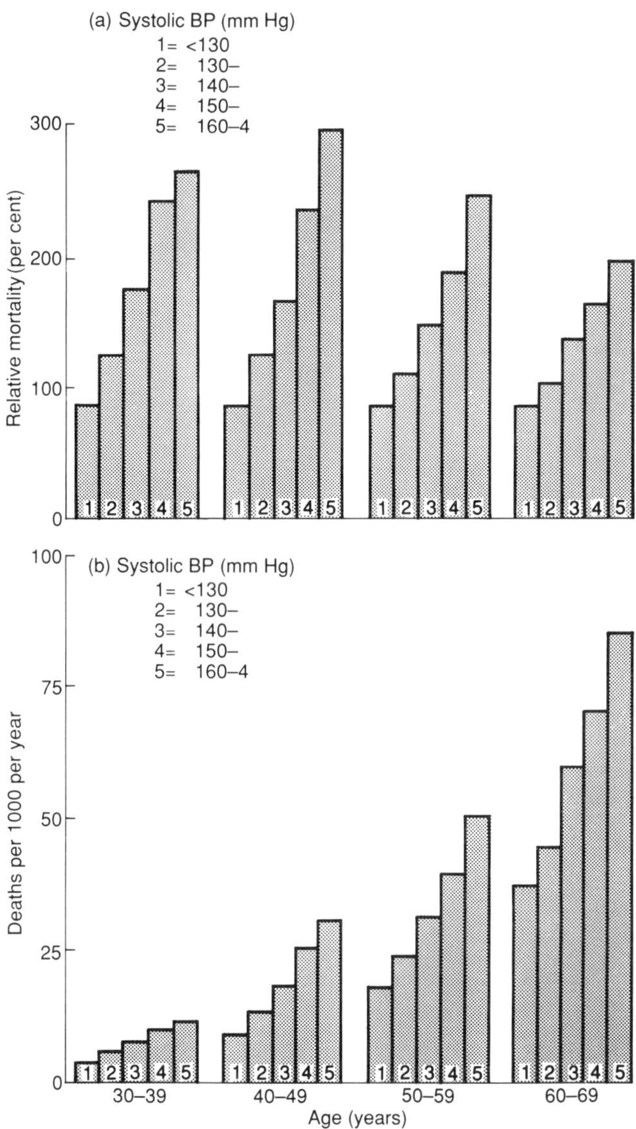

Fig. 14.2 Age-specific mortality in men according to blood pressure and age, from life insurance data: (a) relative risk; (b) absolute risk. (From Rose 1981)

Absolute risk

Of much more significance to the individual patients and their doctors, however, is their absolute risk of dying or developing a cardiovascular complication in the foreseeable future. Absolute risks are much greater in older patients (Fig. 14.2b).

Data about the absolute risk of untreated blood pressure are based on information obtained before the advent of the effective hypertenive therapy. The two-year survival rate for malignant hypertension is around 10 per cent, and patients with a diastolic blood pressure above 130 mmHg have a 40 per cent two-year survival rate if left untreated. Moderate hypertensives with diastolic blood pressures of between 110 and 129 mmHg have an 80 per cent two-year survial rate. Patients with mild hypertension, however (DBP 90–105 mmHg), who have been included in more recent clinical trials have a mortality rate of only 1.5 per cent per annum.

Combined risk

The significance of a particular level of high blood pressure is also greatly influenced by the presence or absence of other risk factors. The multiplicative risks of combining high blood pressure with raised serum cholesterol and smoking are shown in Fig. 15.11. Impaired glucose tolerance, and evidence of arterial disease or end-organ damage are more powerful risk factors. It is possible to combine these factors into a score that will predict an individual's risk of developing chronic heart disease in the next five years (Fig. 14.3).

Attributable risk

The problem facing the epidemiologist concerned not just for the individual patient but for the prevention of arterial disease in the whole population, is that while there are a small number of patients with moderate or severe hypertension or multiple risk factors, there is a very much larger group of patients with moderately elevated risks in whom the majority of cardiovascular events will occur. Taking high blood pressure alone, two-thirds of the attributable coronary deaths and three-quarters of the attributable deaths or strokes occur in men with diastolic pressure below 100 mmHg. Even using the multiple risk factor score only about half of all coronary events will occur in the fifth of patients with the highest scores.

The benefits of treatment of high blood pressure

The benefits of treatment of very high blood pressure were clearly established in the Veteran's Administration trials in the 1960s. In these trials, there were

1 Number of years smoking	×7.5 =	
2 Doctor diagnosis of heart disease	+265	
3 Doctor diagnosis of diabetes	+150	
4 Current angina	+150	
5 Either parent died from heart trouble	+80	
6 Systolic blood pressure	×4.5	
	Total score	

Score	Risk of heart attack in next five years (Men aged 40–60)
< 690	1:250
690–804	1:100
805–889	1:40
890–999	1:30
> 1000	1:10

Fig. 14.3 Combined score for heart attack risk. (Based on data from Shaper *et al.* 1986)

clear benefits of treatment in prevention vascular events for those with a diastolic blood pressure of 115 mmHg or more (Veteran's Administration 1967).

Subsequently, a large number of trials have investigated the benefits of treatment at lower levels of blood pressure. Individually, these trials have shown clear benefits from treatment of those with diastolic blood pressure of 105 mmHg or more in reduction of stroke and heart failure, but inconclusive evidence of benefit in reduction of coronary heart disease risk. But a meta-analysis of trials which have included patients with diastolic blood pressure less than 110 mmHg has shown reduction in stroke events of about one-third and of coronary heart disease events of almost one-quarter over five years associated with a reduction in diastolic pressure of 5 mmHg (Collins *et al.* 1990).

Until recently, all hypertension trials were based on diastolic blood pressure and ignored systolic pressure. Isolated systolic blood pressure is a better predictor than diastolic blood pressure of vascular events and should therefore not be ignored even though guidance on treatment cannot be based on trial evidence.

Older patients have a higher absolute risk of cardiovascular events. But early hypertension trials excluded those over 65 years and only recently have a few trials investigated the benefits of treatment in the older age group.

These trials indicate that treatment of systolic blood pressure of 160 mmHg or over or diastolic blood pressure of 115 mmHg or more in those aged 65–74 years results in substantial reduction in stroke risk (MRC 1992).

Hypertension screening in practice

Every practice should formulate a policy and protocol for hypertension screening and management. This should be part of overall cardiovascular risk assessment and management; blood pressure screening alone, although common in the past, is inappropriate. It should always take account of personal and family history, should be accompanied by enquiry and advice about lifestyle (especially smoking, diet, alcohol consumption, and exercise habits) and by consideration of the need to exclude hyperlipidaemia.

A simple screening protocol such as that based on the 'three-box system' (Fig. 14.4) should be established. The practice nurse has a major role in screening, and it has been shown that a systematic approach involving practice nurses can achieve substantial improvement in ascertainment.

1. those with moderate or severe hypertension justifying treatment in is own right;
2. patients with mild hypertension which is contributing to their oveall cardiovascular risk;
3. the remainder of the practice population.

Moderate or severe hypertension

This is the small group of patients who are at substantial risk from their high blood pressure alone and will benefit significantly from treatment. The evidence suggests that the cut-off point of diastolic blood pressure 105 mmHg or more in younger patients and 110 mmHg or more in those over age 65 would be an appropriate definition for this group.

They will be detected by a policy of measuring every patient's blood pressure every five years, and those with mild hypertension every year.

Their management should include non-pharmacological methods of reducing blood pressure, which may or may not be sufficient, vigorous attention to other risk factors, and appropriate education and reinforcement to encourage compliance with the treatment.

Mild hypertension

This much more substantial group has diastolic blood pressures of between 90 and 105 mmHg. If repeated measurements over three to four months

Target
20–80 years (priority 35–64 years) especially where clinically indicated, e.g. family history, hypertension

Method
Large cuff (13″×5″)
DBP phase V
Action based on minimum of 3 readings

Three-box system

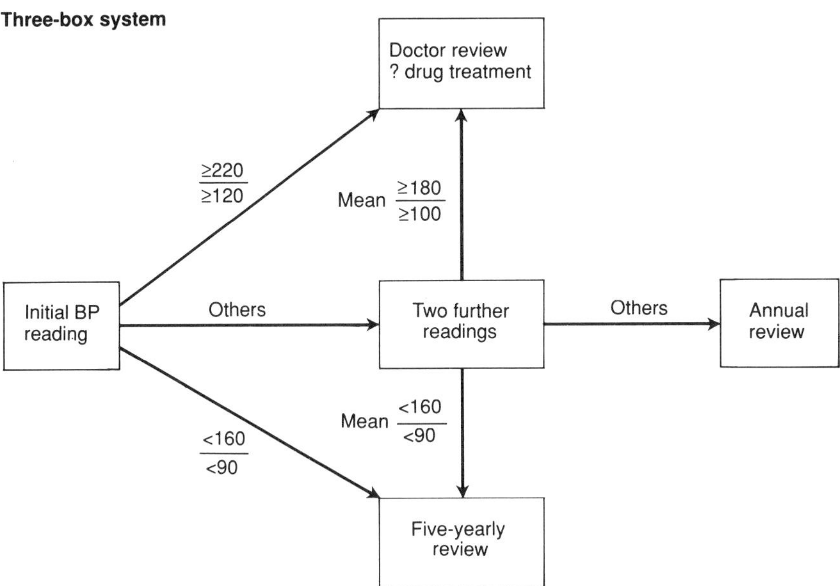

Treatment
Non-pharmacological: weight ↓, alcohol ↓
Drug treatment threshold: diastolic 100
But flexibility {age
{other risk factors
Attention to other risk factors especially smoking, lipids

Fig. 14.4 Blood pressure screening protocol.

show that the blood pressure is sustained at this level, they should receive a full assessment, as the significance of their high blood pressure alone is greatly influenced by the presence of other risk factors or evidence of end-organ damage. They should all receive advice about the reduction of weight, alcohol intake, and other risk factors and treatment should be reserved for those at increased risk. They require at least annual follow-up.

The practice population

If the distribution of blood pressures in the whole population could be reduced the impact of the small benefit for a large number of patients would be as significant as the benefits of detecting and treating those patients who are at a high risk. The objectives should include achievement of optimal body weight (body mass index, BMI, less than 25); restriction of alcohol intake (less than 21 units weekly for men and 14 units weekly for women), moderation of salt intake (by avoiding salty foods and not adding salt to food in cooking or at the table), and regular moderate exercise (for example, half an hour of brisk walking two or three times a week) should all be encouraged. There is also evidence that regular relaxation can lower blood pressure (see Chapter 13).

Summary

- High blood pressure is an independent risk factor for cardiovascular disease—stroke, myocardial infarction, and heart failure.
- Treatment of patients with a diastolic blood pressure of 110 mmHg or greater confers substantial benefits in reducing cardiovascular risk.
- Treatment of patients with a diastolic blood pressure of 90–110 mmHg also confers benefits in reducing the risk of stroke in particular, but also coronary heart disease.
- Lifestyle changes—avoidance of smoking, limitation of alcohol intake, weight control, and exercise are beneficial.
- All those less than age 80 years will benefit from treatment, though in the older age group particular attention should be paid to overall cardiovascular risk, and possible adverse effects of pharmacological treatment deserves special consideration.
- Assessment and management of hypertension should always be part of a multifactorial risk approach.

References

Collins, R., Peto, R., MacMahon, S., Hebert, P., Fiebach, N. H., Eberlein, K. A., *et al.* (1990). Blood pressure, stroke and coronary heart disease. *Lancet*, **335**, 827–38.

MacMahon, S., Peto, R., Cutler, J., Collins, R., Sorlie, P., Neaton, J., *et al.* (1990). Blood pressure, stroke and coronary heart disease. *Lancet*, **335**, 765–74.

Marmot, M. E. (1986). Epidemiology and the art of the soluble. *The Lancet*, **i**, 897–900.

Medical Research Council (1992). MRC trial of treatment of hypertension in older adults: principal results. *Brit. Med. J.*, **304**, 405–12.

Rose, G. (1981). Strategy of prevention: lessons from cardiovascular disease. *British Medical Journal*, **282**, 1847–51.

Shaper, A. E., Pocock, S. J., Phillips, A. N., and Walker, M. (1986). Identifying men at high risk of heart attacks: strategy for use in general practice. *British Medical Journal*, **293**, 474–9.

Veteran's Administration Study Group. (1967). Effects of treatment on morbidity in hypertension: results in patients with diastolic blood pressures averaging 115 through 129 mmHg. *J. Am. Med. Ass.*, **202**, 116.

Further reading

British Medical Journal (1987). *ABC of hypertension*, British Medical Association, London.

Hasler, J. C. and Schofield, T. P. C. (1990). *Continuing care in general practice*, 2nd edn. Oxford University Press.

15 Prevention of cardiovascular disease

Godfrey Fowler

Diseases of the circulatory system account for over 40 per cent of all deaths in Britain (Fig. 15.1). This is by far the largest cause of death and compares with less than a quarter caused by cancer.

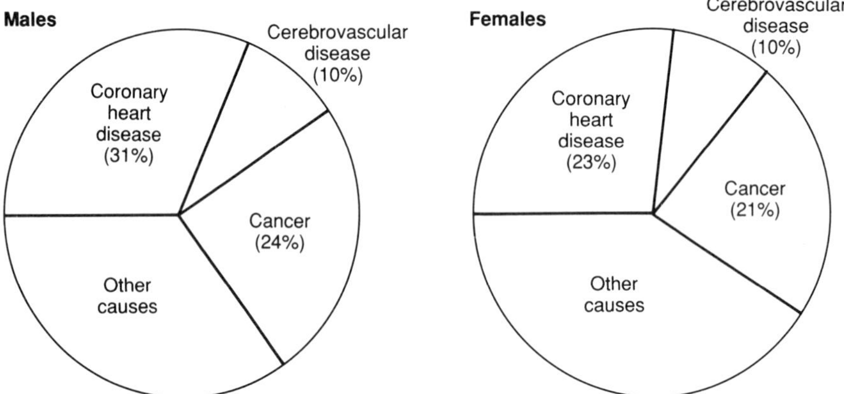

Fig. 15.1 Overall causes of death in the UK as a percentage of the total, 1985. (Data from OPCS.)

Coronary heart disease

Coronary heart disease (CHD) is the single most common cause of death, accounting for about 180 000 deaths a year in the UK, over one-quarter of all deaths. The international 'league table' of CHD deaths shows all UK countries at or near the top (Fig. 15.2). Having risen steeply over the previous 50 years, coronary heart disease mortality reached a peak in Britain in the late 1970s and has since shown a small decline. This peak was reached about ten years earlier in some countries, notably the USA and Australia, and the decline there has been much steeper—almost one-third over the last two decades (Figs. 15.3 and 15.4).

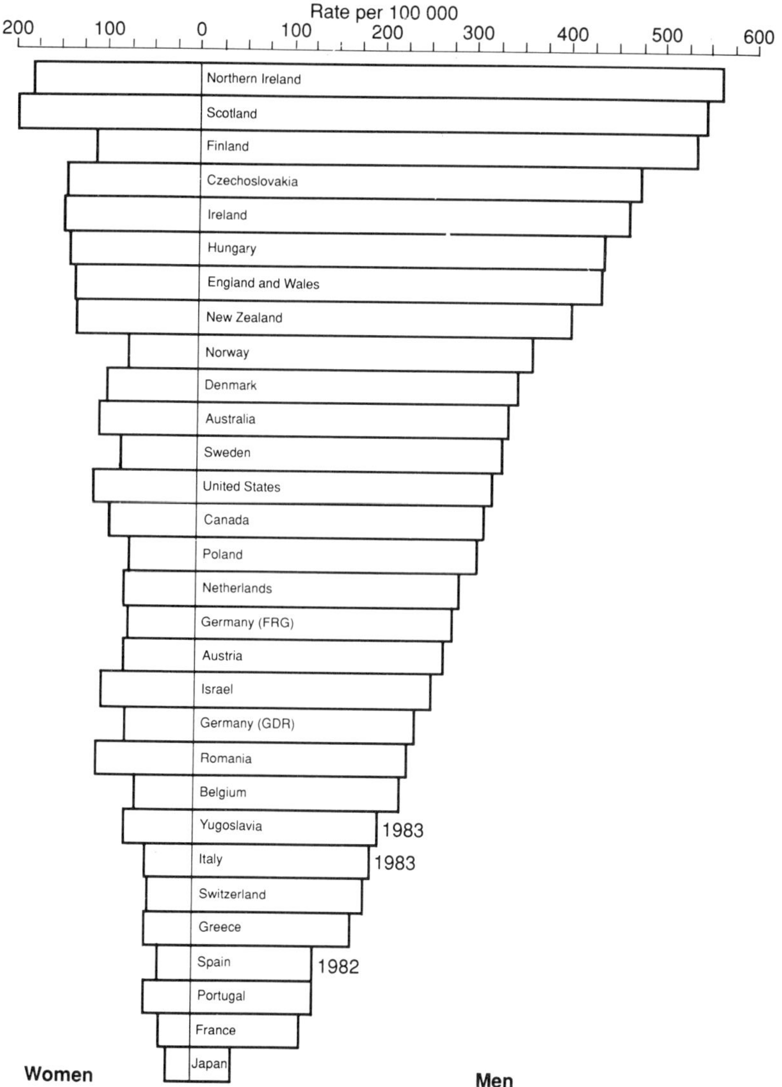

Fig. 15.2 Coronary heart disease mortality rates for men and women aged 40–69. Age-standardized rates per 100 000 for 1985 unless otherwise stated. (Data from Cardiovascular Epidemiology Unit, Dundee.)

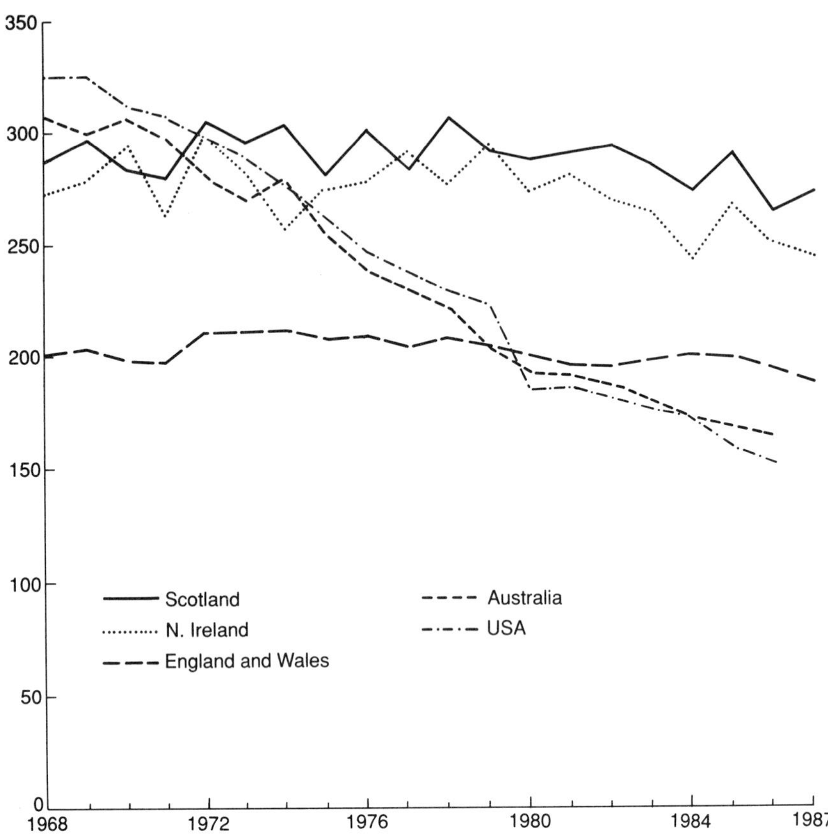

Fig. 15.3 Death rates from coronary heart disease by country for 1968–87 (for women aged 35–74). (From WHO statistics in Coronary Prevention Group/British Heart Foundation 1988)

Risk factors

Many epidemiological studies, such as the Framington study in the USA and British Regional Heart Study in the UK, have established risk factors for coronary heart disease. These risk factors are conditions associated with coronary heart disease and which have been established, with varying degrees of certainty, to have a causal relationship to it.

Family history of cardiovascular disease at an early age is an important risk factor. Although not amenable to change, it indicates those in whom attention to modifiable risk factors is especially important.

Other risk factors which are important but likewise not amenable to

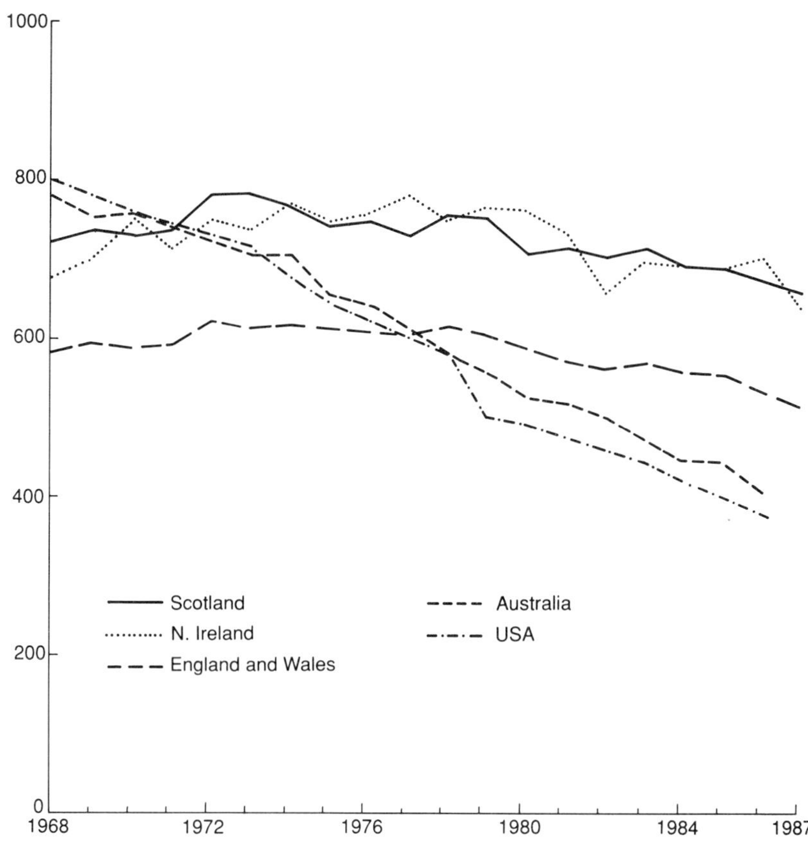

Fig. 15.4 Death rates from coronary heart disease by country for 1968–87 (for men aged 35–74). (From WHO statistics in Coronary Prevention Group/British Heart Foundation 1988)

change are age and male sex, the risk of coronary heart disease increasing with age and being greater for men than for women, especially in the younger age group.

Three alterable risk factors have been shown to be strongly and consistently associated with the development of the disease. Their avoidance or reversal has, in some measure, been shown to reduce the risk of the disease. They also seem biologically plausible. The *three major risk factors* are:

- raised blood lipids;
- high blood pressure;
- cigarette smoking.

There is accumulating evidence that thrombotic factors, especially the level of fibrinogen, may also be important.

Other modifiable risk factors that appear to have a weaker influence but are important nevertheless include:

- physical inactivity;
- obesity;
- psychosocial factors.

Diabetes is an important risk factor: diabetics have twice the coronary heart disease mortality of non-diabetics.

Finally, a history of previous cardiovascular disease in an individual is, perhaps not surprisingly, an important risk factor for coronary heart disease.

Blood lipids

High blood cholesterol appears to be the key risk factor. It is an essential and sufficient risk factor and the two other major risk factors, high blood pressure and smoking, appear not to exert their influence when cholesterol levels are low.

In the Seven Countries study, initiated in the 1950s, Keys demonstrated a clear relationship between the mean cholesterol levels in population samples of middle-aged men in seven countries (Finland, Greece, Holland, Italy, Japan, USA, Yugoslavia) and their subsequent coronary heart disease incidence and mortality (Fig. 15.5). Many subsequent studies have shown a correlation between the mean serum cholesterol levels of communities and their rates of coronary heart disease.

Within communities, epidemiological studies, such as follow-up of the multiple risk factor intervention trial (MRFIT) screenees, have also shown a correlation between cholesterol levels and coronary heart disease risk (Fig. 15.6).

Intervention trials aimed at lowering serum cholesterol and testing the effect of this on coronary heart disease risk have, however, not been as conclusive as anticipated. One limitation on such trials is the extent to which it is reasonable to expect reversal of atherosclerotic changes in a relatively short time in middle-aged people, when it has taken decades to develop. Many such trials have been multifactorial, concerned with other coronary heart disease risk factors as well as cholesterol. Although these trials have often been interpreted as disappointing in terms of reductions achieved, collectively they provide evidence that lowering cholesterol levels by diet (supplemented in some trials by medication) can reduce coronary heart disease mortality. But there is still debate about the effect on all-causes mortality, especially about whether very low cholesterol levels cause increased risk of death from cancer and other causes.

Total cholesterol is the basic measurement of serum lipids. The major

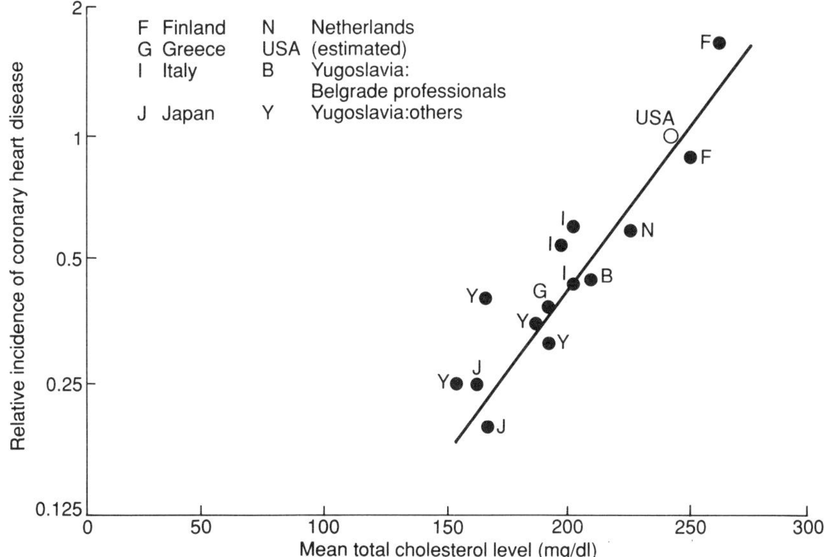

Fig. 15.5 Serum cholesterol level and incidence of new coronary heart disease (any type) in different populations and subgroups. (Note: 1 mmol/l ≈ 38.6 mg/dl.) (After Keys 1980)

atherogenic influence seems to be exerted through low-density lipoprotuin (LDL) cholesterol which constitutes about two-thirds of the total, the remainder being mostly high-density cholesterol (HDL) which has a protective effect. Total serum cholesterol provides the simplest and most useful lipid measurement for screening purposes. Measurement of HDL and triglycerides may be useful in decisions on management of those with hyperlipidaemia particularly in women and especially in influencing decisions about drug treatment.

In studies of populations, coronary heart disease mortality increases progressively with a cholesterol level above about 5 mmol/l. The mean level of cholesterol in the British population is about 6 mmol/l, a level associated with about a twofold increase in coronary heart disease mortality compared with those with levels of 5 mmol or less.

High blood pressure

As with lipids, many epidemiological studies have demonstrated a correlation between blood pressure and coronary heart disease risk; systolic pressure appears to be as important as diastolic pressure. However, this association between high blood pressure and coronary heart disease risk occurs only in populations that have mean high blood cholesterol levels.

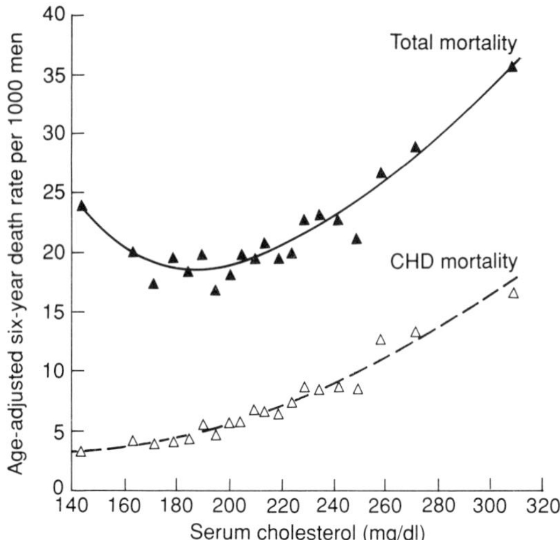

Fig. 15.6 Age-adjusted six-year CHD and total mortality per 1000 men screened for MRFIT according to serum cholesterol. The entire cohort of 361 662 men was divided into aproximate twentieths, and each point represents the mortality (either CHD or total) and the mean cholesterol level in one of those twentieths. Hand-fitted lines are drawn through the points. (From Martin *et al.* 1986)

There is now clear evidence that lowering blood pressure reduces coronary heart disease risk, and even better evidence that it reduces the risk of stroke and heart failure (Fig. 15.7).

Cigarette smoking

In countries and communities with high mean cholesterol levels there is also a strong correlation between cigarette smoking and coronary heart disease morbidity and mortality (Fig. 15.8). The relative risk when compared with non-smokers is about two but is greater in the younger age group. In women, smoking increases the risk of coronary heart disease associated with oral contraception, at least in older women.

There is good evidence that stopping smoking reduces coronary heart disease risk relatively quickly, half the excess risk disappearing in the first year or two after stopping smoking.

Family history

Family history of cardiovascular disease, especially at an early age, is an important risk factor for coronary heart disease. In the majority, family

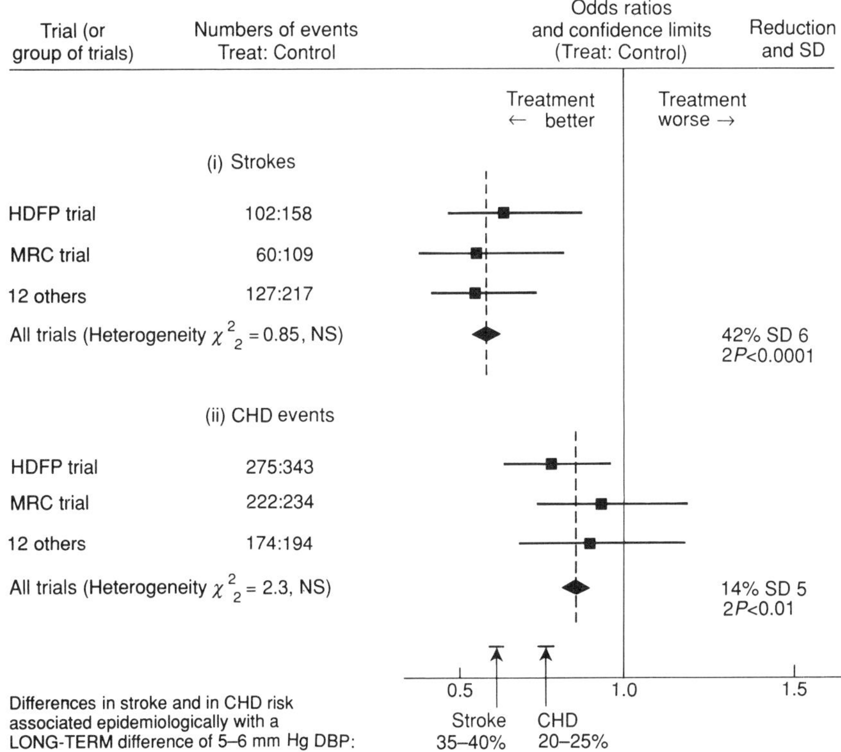

Fig. 15.7 Reduction in the odds of stroke and of coronary heart disease in the HDFP trial, the MRC trial, and in all 12 other smaller unconfounded randomized trials of anti-hypertensive therapy (mean DBP differences 5–6 mmHg for five years). Full squares represent the simple odds ratio for the two larger trials and the properly stratified odds ratio for the combination of the 12 smaller trials (sizes of squares are proportional to number of events and 95% cls for estimates of relative risk are denoted by vertical lines). (From MacMahon *et al.* 1990)

history implies a mixture of genetic and environmental influences. In a small proportion of people, family history is the result of genetically determined 'familial hypercholesterolaemia'; this occurs in the heterozygous form in about one in 500 of the population and in the homozygous form very rarely.

The importance of family history is in identifying those in whom attention to amenable risk factors may be particularly fruitful.

Physical inactivity

Several studies have investigated the relationship between physical activity and coronary heart disease risk. In a study of British civil servants, vigorous

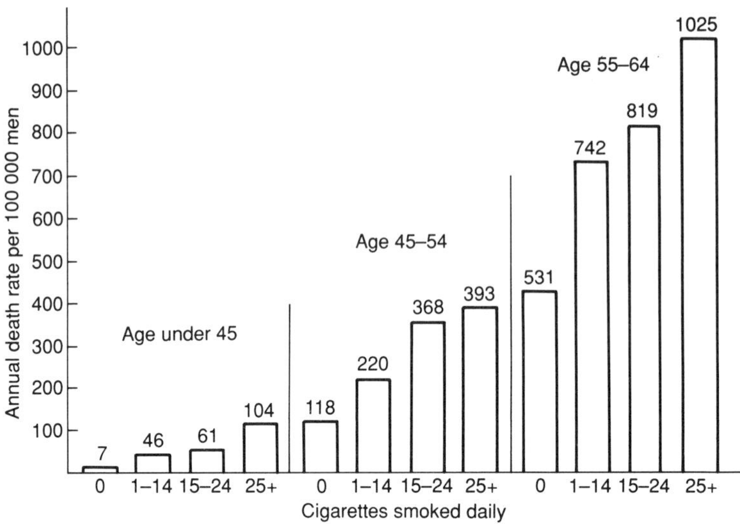

Fig. 15.8 British Doctors Study: mortality from coronary heart disease in male non-smokers and current smokers by age and smoking category. With rising age the relative risk to smokers compared with non-smokers gets less, although the number of deaths associated with smoking increases. (From Royal College of Physicians 1977)

leisure time activity was found to protect against coronary heart disease morbidity and mortality. Studies in the USA similarly showed that dockers engaged in more strenuous activities than other of their colleagues had lower coronary heart disease mortality.

There is now general agreement that general physical activity, whether in work or in leisure, is protective against coronary heart disease risk (see Chapter 13).

Obesity

Being overweight is associated with an increased risk of coronary heart disease, but also with increased levels of serum cholesterol and blood pressure as well as decreased levels of physical activity. When account is taken of these risk factors associated with obesity, the latter appears not to have an independent effect.

This does not mean that being overweight is unimportant in relation to coronary heart disease. It is a 'visible target' and may be seen as a proxy for other risk factors.

Psycho-social factors

The public generally regards stress as an important contributor to coronary heart disease, but the evidence relating stress and psychological factors to coronary heart disease is poor.

Early studies (from the USA) of behaviour in relation to coronary heart disease indicated that type A personalities, characterized by aggressiveness and competitiveness, were more prone to coronary heart disease than the more phlegmatic type B individuals. Subsequent studies have cast doubt on these findings.

Other studies suggest that coronary heart disease risk factors can be modified by relaxation.

It seems likely that psychological factors do play a significant part, although it is difficult to study their influence (see Chapter 12).

Socio-economic factors are important in relation to coronary heart disease. Coronary heart disease mortality is higher in lower socio-economic groups and the gap has widened in the last decade. Only part of this difference between upper and lower socio-economic classes is explained by differences in levels of the major risk factors (Fig. 15.9). (See also Chapter 3.)

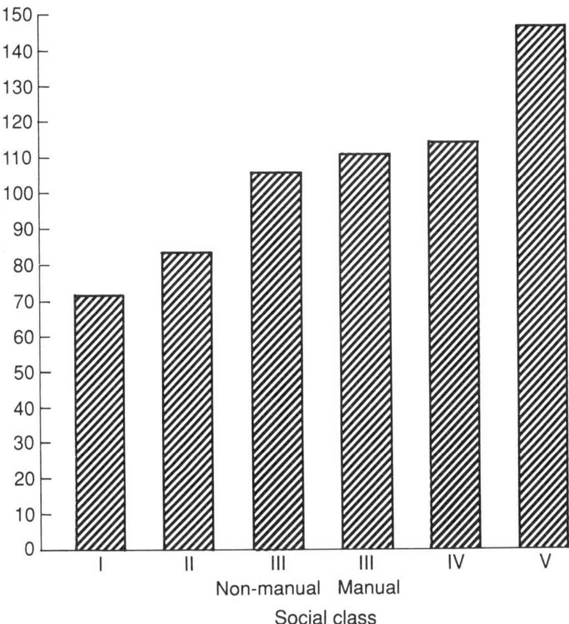

Fig. 15.9 Standard mortality ratios for coronary heart disease for males aged 20–64 years, England and Wales 1979–83. (Data from OPCS 1986)

The scope for prevention

The evidence relating risk factors to coronary heart disease provides the basis for prevention. Avoidance or reversal of the risks should lead to avoidance or reduction in the disease, but there are two important considerations.

1. Although those with the highest levels of risk factors are collectively at greatest risk, this risk is not equally shared amongst these individuals. This may be illustrated by taking adult men aged 40–55 years who are at risk from being in the top 20 per cent of cholesterol and blood pressures. Half the coronary heart disease events occurring in all adult men in this age group will occur in this 20 per cent, two-thirds of who who will nevertheless remain well over the next 25 years. So, although prediction of risk for the group is reasonably strong, that for individuals is weak.

   The interaction of risk factors (Fig. 15.10) is particularly important and this can be illustrated from the MRFIT data (Fig. 15.11). This interaction is the basis of various CHD risk scores such as that based on the British Regional Heart Study data (see Table 15.1).

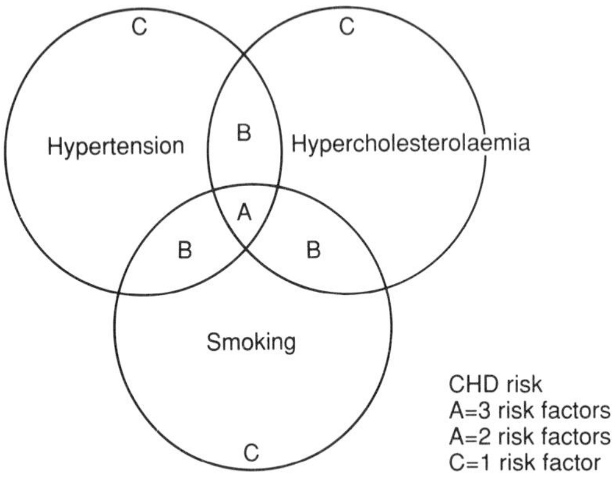

Fig. 15.10 Venn diagram of coronary heart disease risk sets based on three risk factors.

2. Although those with highest levels of risk factors are at greater risk than those with lower levels, they are fewer in number. Therefore, in absolute numbers more coronary heart disease deaths occur in those who have 'normal levels' of risk factors who are much more numerous. This is illustrated in Fig. 15.12.

Taking 1000 men age 55–64 years, 16 CHD deaths will occur in the 600 or so who have cholesterol levels below 6.5 mmol/l and 10 in the 100 or so who

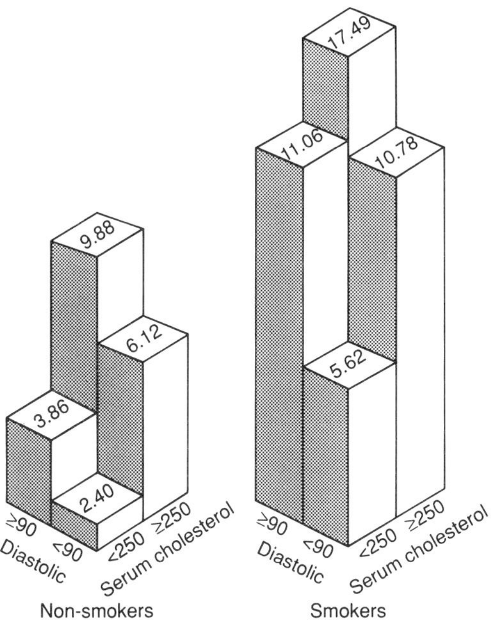

Fig. 15.11 Five-year age-adjusted coronary heart disease death rates/1000 for 325 384 white males aged 35–57 screened for the MRFIT programme, by smoking habit, diastolic blood pressure, and serum cholesterol level (in mg/dl). (From Marmot 1986)

have cholesterol levels above 7.5 mmol/l. A prevention strategy aimed at both the group at high relative risk and also the majority of the population at lower risk is therefore essential.

The approach to the majority of the population depends on community education to modify lifestyle especially that with respect to smoking and diet, aimed at a reduction in the level of risk factors in the population as a whole. Programmes such as the North Karelia and Stanford projects have been concerned with testing these approaches.

In addition to this, special help for the high-risk group depends on their identification by screening and a more intensive effort at lifestyle changes, coupled with identification and management of high levels of blood pressure and lipids, including consideration of drug treatment.

The role of primary health care

National Health Service general practice in Britain is uniquely placed both to participate in a population approach to coronary heart disease prevention

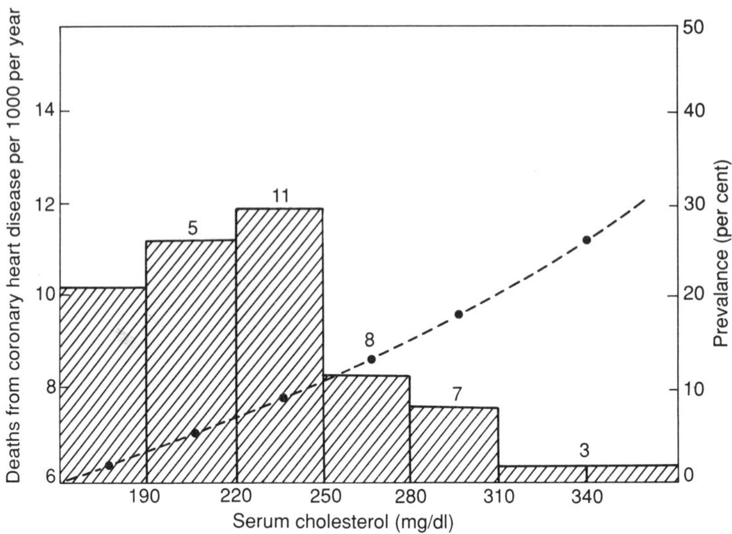

Fig. 15.12 Prevalence distribution of serum cholestorol concentration related to coronary heart disease mortality (broken curve) in men aged 55–64. The number above each bar represents an estimate of attributable deaths per 1000 population per 10 years. (Note: 1 mmol/l ≈ 38.6 mg/dl.) (Based on the Framingham study, from Rose 1981)

and to identify and help those at high risk. Health education and health promotion are becoming more prominent feaures of general practice and are now included in the 'Terms of service' of NHS general practitioners (see the Appendix).

About three-quarters of the population has contact with general practice every year and the average person has three or four such annual contacts. The primary purpose of these patient-initiated contacts is generally the management of symptomatic illness, but they also provide an opportunity for:

- health education and promotion;
- screening on an opportunistic basis.

There is evidence that patients increasingly expect doctors to enquire and advise about aspects of lifestyle, such as diet and smoking.

Although research on helping patients to stop smoking shows that simple advice given in general practice is effective, surveys of medical records generally indicate a low level of recording of such things as smoking habit, weight and dietary issues, and alcohol consumption. Thus, a large gap exists between potential and achievement.

The potential–achievement gap

The reasons for this potential–achievement gap include:

1. the demand-orientated philosophy of medical care;
2. the brevity of general practice consultations;
3. the workload;
4. the lack of a coordinated, systematic approach;
5. the need for a team approach.

One method which has been found successful in achieving a higher level of involvement of general practice in preventive care depends on the employment of practice nurses in a preventive role (see Chapter 4).

Recommendations for action

- *Government* should encourage and facilitate the adoption of a healthy lifestyle by the population through educational, economic, and other measures. Influences on the tobacco and food industries are of key importance.
- *The media, schools, and other education bodies*, industrial organizations, and health institutions and authorities all have important contributions to make to a coronary heart disease prevention programme.
- *Doctors (in both community and hospital)* should be involved in developing and implementing national and local programmes of health education concerned with reducing coronary heart disease risk in the population as a whole.

Apart from a role in this population approach, general practice teams have a particular opportunity to identify and help individuals at special risk. This means the adoption of some form of screening and the most appropriate one is an opportunistic approach in adults, using patient-initiated contacts (see Box 15.1).

Patients in whom blood cholesterol should be measured include those with:

- personal history or signs of coronary heart disease or diabetes, or any stigmata of hyperlipidaemia;
- strong family history of coronary heart disease (first-degree relative, male < 50, female < 55) or of hyperlipidaemia;
- multiple risk factors (a 'risk scoring' system may be used to identify, for example, those in the top 20 per cent a risk with a 1 in 10 likelihood of a CHD event within five years).

This information should be recorded in the notes in an easily accessible form. This may be on a special risk factor record card such as that illustrated in

Box 15.1: Opportunistic screening

This should consist of the following:

- Enquiry about cardiovascular disease and deaths in first degree relatives, especially a an early age (<50 years men, <55 years women).
- Enquiry about a personal history of cardiovascular disease or diabetes.
- Measurement of blood pressure and careful assessment if this is raised.
- Measurement of weight and height, calculation of body mass index (see Chapter 10).
- Enquiry about smoking habit and appropriate advice.
- Enquiry about diet and alcohol consumption, with appropriate advice.
- Measurement of random total serum cholesterol selectively in those at high risk because of other factors.
- Measurement of blood sugar in those seriously obese.

Fig. 15.13. The aim should be to achieve at least one risk factor assessment in every adult patient every five years. Ideally, the age-group 20–65 years should be targeted but if this prospect seems overwhelming, start with the 35–65 year age-group, or even just those aged 40–60 years.

Management of risk factors

Guidelines of the management of various risk factors are shown in Box 15.2.

Implementation of these recommendations

Implementation of these recommendations will generally depend on a team approach. Systematic case finding using an opportunistic method of recruitment can be achieved by practice nurses (Chapter 4). Management of risk factors can be shared between doctors and nurses on an agreed basis.

Cerebrovascular disease

Incidence

'Stroke' is the third most common cause of death (after coronary heart disease and cancer). About 100 000 people have a stroke each year in Britain

Box 15.2: Management of risk factors

Blood pressure

- Those with sustained levels at, or above, 180/100 justify active management and consideration of drug treatment.
- Those with a level of 160/90 or less should be reviewed five yearly.
- Those with blood pressures between these levels should be reviewed annually (see Chapter 14).

Weight

- Those with a body mass index greater than 25 require dietary advice and supervision (Chapter 10).

Smoking

- Those who are smokers should be given simple verbal and written advice and offered support (see Chapter 9).

Cholesterol

- Although the aim is to achieve cholesterol levels below 5.2 mmol/l, dietary advice should be focused particularly on those with levels above 6.5 mmol/l and on those with other risk factors. Those with levels above 7.8 mmol/l warrant consideration of drug treatment as well as dietary advice, especially where there are other risk factors.

and there are about 50000 stroke-related deaths; many survivors suffer severe disabilty. Stroke incidence has been declining, at least since the 1950s; reliable data before that date are not available.

Stroke is caused by a vascular event which results in loss of perfusion. Basically, there are three types of such vascular event: thrombosis, embolism, and haemorrhage. Thrombosis and embolism result in infarction. Haemorrhage may be intracerebral or subarachnoid. The age-specific incidence and proportion of each stroke type by age (male and female combined) from one study are illustrated in Figs. 15.14 and 15.15.

Risk factors

The risk factors for stroke and the strength of the causal relationship is shown in Table 15.1.

Age and sex

The *Royal College of Physicians report on stroke* showed that the incidence of strokes increased rapidly over the age of 55, so in those aged 85 and over it

HEALTH SUMMARY

Name **MALE**

D.O.B.		SMWD		No.	

Own Occupation
Partner's Occupation

Date	Date	Date	
1st B/P	2nd B/P	3rd B/P	Mean if applicable

Weight	Ideal Weight	Height

Nutrition advice	Exercise

Smoker	Cigarettes	Pipe	Since 19
Non Smoker	Never	Stopped 19	

Family History of CVA or MI

Diabetes	Yes	Insulin	OHD	Diet
	No			

Date of Tetanus	1st	2nd	3rd	Booster

Urine Date	Protein	Sugar

Alcohol

Notes Advice given Further action

Fig. 15.13 Risk factors record card.

was 40 per 1000, (Fig. 15.15), although in the Oxford Community Stroke Study, it was only 20 per 1000 in this age group.

Stroke is more common in men than in women, though the sex difference is much less marked than for coronary heart disease, the rate in men being rather less than twice that in women.

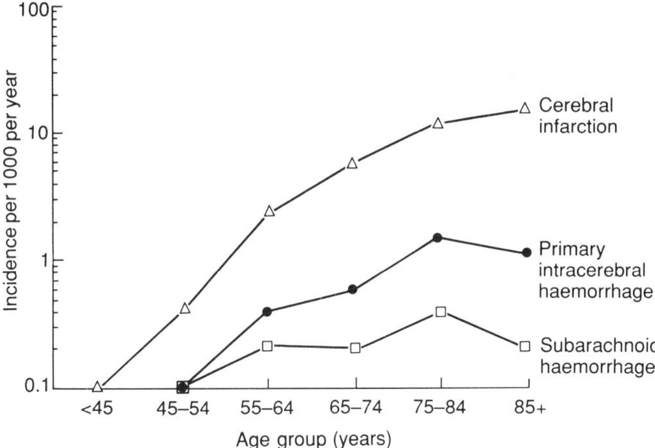

Fig. 15.14 The age-specific annual incidence of pathological types of first-ever stroke, male and female combined (note logarithmic scale). (From Bamford *et al.* 1990)

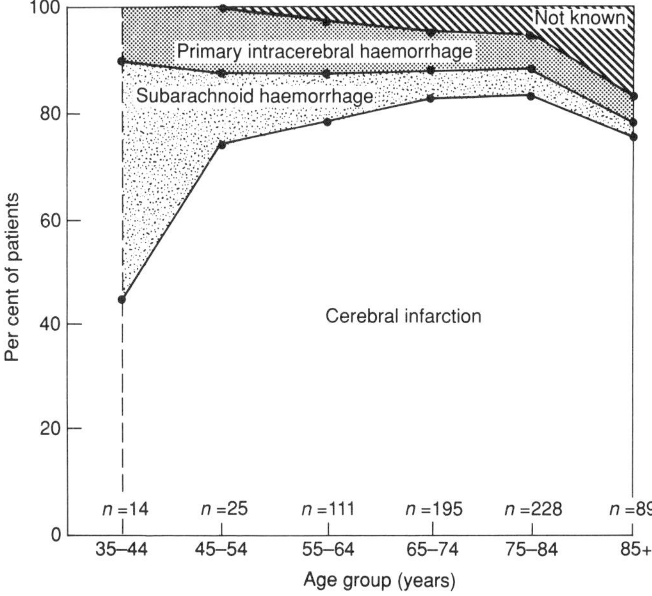

Fig. 15.15 The proportion of each stroke type by age (male and female combined). (From Bamford *et al.* 1990)

Table 15.1 Risk factors for stroke

Risk factors for stroke	Strength of causal association
Increasing age	††††
Hypertension	††††
Male sex	†††
Existing vascular disease	†††
Cardiac dysfunction	†††
Diabetes	†††
Smoking	††
Alcohol intake	††
High lipids	††
High fibrinogen	†
High haemotocrit	†
Geography	†
Family history	†
Obesity	†

Hypertension

Apart from age, the outstandingly important risk factor for stroke is high blood pressure. A number of epidemiological studies have demonstrated clear relationships between both systolic and diastolic blood pressure and stroke incidence.

Many randomized trials have also demonstrated that lowering blood pressure reduces stroke incidence, both in middle age and in the elderly (at least up to the age of 80 years). The effect of treatment on risk reduction in those with mild hypertension (phase V diastolic 90–109 mmHg) in the 35–64 year age-group is illustrated (Table 15.2).

To what extent the decline in stroke deaths this century is due to detection and treatment of hypertension is debatable, though it is thought such treatment probably accounts for a minority of the reduction.

Heart disease

Heart disease is associated with an increase risk of stroke, and atrial fibrillation carries a particularly high relative risk (and is present in a substantial proportion of stroke patients, particularly the elderly).

Ischaemic heart disease, sino-atrial disease, valvular disease (inluding prostheic values), bacterial endocarditis, and cardiac failure all increase stroke risk.

Table 15.2 The number of patients to be treated for five yars to prevent one stroke, according to entry diastolic pressure and age. (MRC trial data, from Miall and Greenberg 1988)

Age (years)	Entry DBP	
	<100 mmHg	100–109 mmHg
35–44		500
45–54	400	118
55–64	286	57
35–64	500	95

Conversely, stroke survivors are more likely to die of coronary heart disease than a further stroke.

Smoking

Although smoking is now an acknowledged risk factor for stroke, the relationship is less important than is the case with coronary heart disease or peripheral arteial disease. Meta-analysis of 32 studies of smoking and stroke suggests an overall relative risk associated with smoking of about 1.5, but ranging from about 3 for those under 55 years to 1.1 for those over 75 years. The relative risks for different types of stroke were: cerebral infarction 1.9, cerebral haemorrhage 0.7, and subarachnoid haemorrhage 2.9.

Lipids

Although the relationship between elevated blood lipids and coronary heart disease is well established, the effect on stroke is less clear. But most studies show a positive relationship between raised lipids and cerebrovascular disease. Data from the MRFIT trial showed a positive relationship between raised serum cholesterol and risk of death from nonhaemorrhagic stroke, but an inverse relationship with haemorrhagic stroke (which is, however, rarer).

Obesity

Obesity is related to hypertension, impaired glucose tolerance,and elevated blood lipids; because of these relationships, it is therefore associated with increased stroke risk. But there is no clear evidence that it is an independent risk factor, though waist:hip ratio may be a positive factor.

Alcohol

As with lipids, the relationship between alcohol consumption and stroke is not clear; but there is good evidence that heavy drinking is associated with increased stroke risk and that moderate alcohol consumption may also adversely influence stroke risk, especially that of subarachnoid haemorrhage. High alcohol consumption is associated with hypertension so, as with obesity, some at least of the increased risk is not independent.

Diabetes

Overall, diabetes approximately doubles the risk of stroke and, with the increasing incidence of diabetes in the elderly, the contribution of this disease to stroke in this age group is important.

Blood viscosity, haematocrit and fibrinogen

The effect of these on cerebral blood flow is undoubtedly important, but evidence relating elevations to increased stroke risk remains debatable.

Transient ischaemic attacks

An important risk factor for stroke is a previous transient ischaemic attack and in hospital-based studies up to a third of strokes have been preceded by one of these. There is evidence that anti-platelet treatment with low-dose aspirin can reduce the risk of subsequent stroke in such patients.

Carotid artery disease

In the absence of trial evidence that carotid endarterectomy is beneficial in reducing stroke risk, there is no good case for screening for carotid artery disease, as a risk factor for stroke, by auscultation of the carotid arteries.

Summary

- The important risk factors for coronary heart disease are family history, premature CHD, hyperlipidaemia, hypertension, and cigarette smoking.
- Lowering blood cholesterol, hypertension treatment, and stopping smoking reduce CHD risk.
- Risk factors interact and a multiple risk factor approach to prevention is therefore important.
- Opportunistic screening in primary care can achieve risk factor measurement but management of risk factors must be an essential sequel to this.

- The risk factors for stroke are the same as those for CHD but hypertension is especially important and heart disease is an important risk factor for stroke.

References and further reading

Bamford, J., *et al.* (1990). The Oxfordshire Community Stroke Project. *Journal of Neurology, Neurosurgery and Psychiatry*, **53**, 824–9.

British Cardiac Society (1987). *Coronary disease prevention.* British Cadiac Society, London.

Coronary heart disease. The need for action (1990). Offices of Health Economics, London.

Coronary Prevention Group/British Heart Foundation (1988). *Statistical information on coronary heart disease.* (PG/BHF), London.

Diet and cardiovascular disease (COMA report) (1984). HMSO, London.

Keys, A. (1980). *Seven countries. A multivariate analysis of death and coronary heart disease.* Harvard University Press, Cambridge, MA.

MacMahon, S., *et al.* (1990). Blood pressure, stroke, and coronary heart disease. *The Lancet*, **335**, 765–74.

Marmot, M. E. (1986). Epidemiology and the art of the soluble. *The Lancet*, **i**, 897–900.

Martin, M. J. *et al.* (1986). Serum cholesterol, blood pressure and mortality: implications from a cohort of 361,662 men (MRFIT). *The Lancet*, **ii**, 933–6.

Miall, W. E. and Greenberg, G. (1988). *Mild hypertension: is there pressure to treat?* Cambridge University Press.

Rose, G. (1981). Strategy of prevention: lessions from cardiovascular disease. *British Medical Journal*, **282**, 1847–51.

Royal College of Physicians (1977). *Smoking and health: the third report from the Royal College of Physicians, London.* Pitman, London.

Royal College of Physicians (1983). *Health or smoking?* Pitman, London.

Royal College of General Practitioners (1981). Prevention of arterial disease in general practice. *Report from general practice* No. 19. RCGP, London.

Shaper, A. E., *et al.* (1987). Risk factors for ischaemic heart disease. *Health Trends*, **19**, 3–7.

World Health Organization (19820. *Prevention of coronary heart disease.* WHO, Geneva.

Addresses (for useful literature)

British Heart Foundation
14 Fitzhardinge Street
London W1H 4DH

The Stroke Association
CHSA House
Whitecross Street
London EC1Y 8JJ

Health Education Authority
Hamilton House
Mabledon Place
London WC1H 9TX

Coronary Prevention Group
102 Gloucester Place
London W1H 3PH

16 Prevention of cancer

Joan Austoker and Muir Gray

Cancer: the size of the problem

Over 250 000 new cases of cancer are registered in the UK each year. On the basis of current incidence rates it is estimated that one in three people will develop cancer at some time during their life. More than 70 per cent of all new cases occur in people aged 60 years and over.

Cancer is now responsible for a quarter of all deaths in the UK, with over 162 000 deaths in 1988. Just a few cancers account for more than half of all cancer death (see Fig. 16.1). Lung cancer alone is responsible for 25 per cent of these deaths. The ten most common cancer in males and females are shown in Fig. 16.2. Breast cancer is the commonest cause of female cancer deaths except in Scotland where female lung cancer deaths now exceed those from breast cancer.

Trends in cancer mortality over the past three decades show that, with the exception of stomach cancer, there has been little improvement in mortality rates from all the major cancers. Moreover the reason for the decline in stomach cancer deaths is unknown.

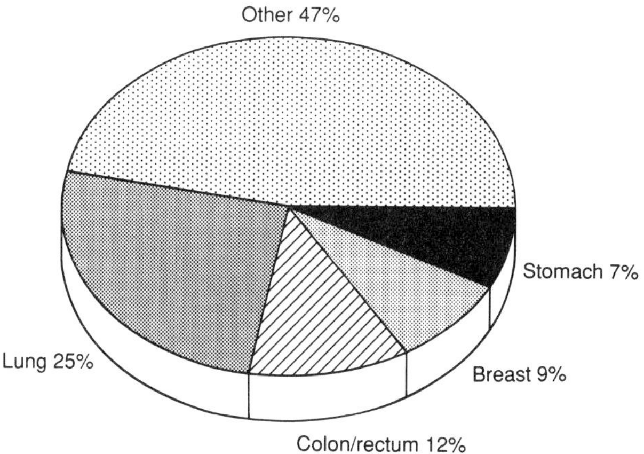

Fig. 16.1 Cancer mortality by site (UK, 1988). Data from the Cancer Research Campaign 1990 Annual Report.

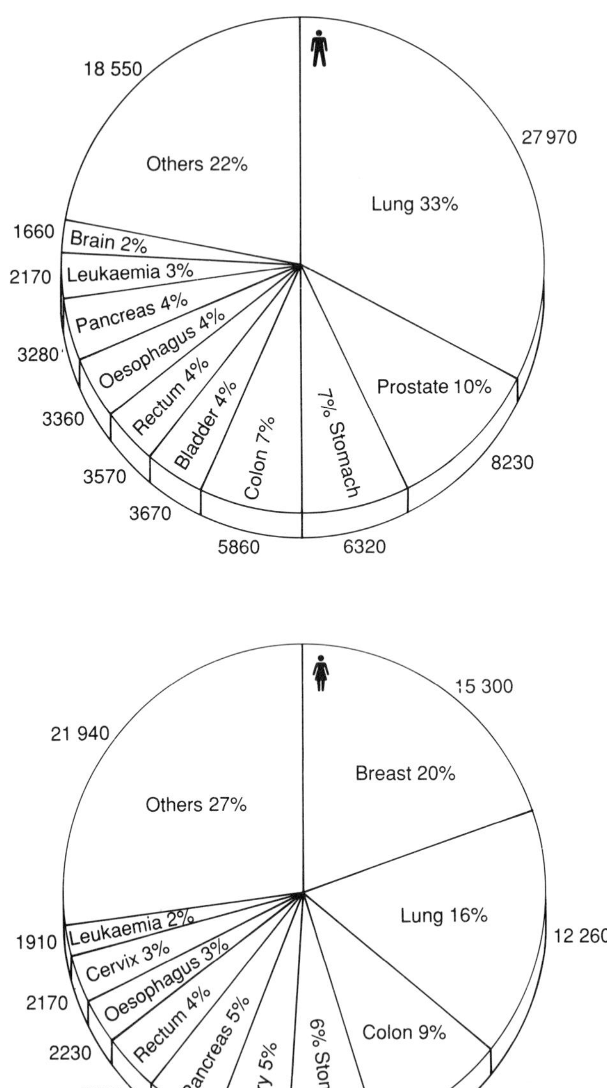

Fig. 16.2 Cancer deaths in the UK, 1988. Data from Cancer Research Campaign 1990 Annual Report.

Cancer prevention: reducing the risk

There is increasing evidence to show that the majority of cancers are potentially avoidable and, moreover, that they could be prevented or diagnosed earlier using knowledge that is already available. The estimated proportion of cancer deaths attributed to various different factors is shown in Fig. 16.3.

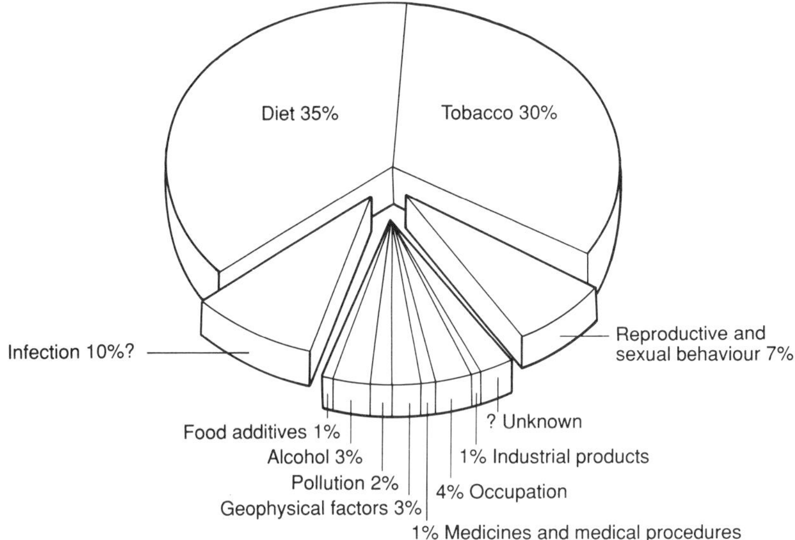

Fig. 16.3 Estimated percentage of cancer deaths attributed to various factors. (Source: Doll and Peto 1981)

At an individual level there is much that can be done to reduce the risk of developing cancer. The age-specific risks are, for the most part, potentially capable of being reduced by at least four-fifths. However, action and positive change is required at many levels to create the conditions under which individuals can realistically make changes to reduce the risks they currently undertake. Primary care teams have a central role in facilitating this process.

The ideal means of effecting cancer control is primary prevention (e.g. avoidance of cigarette smoking). Second best is effective treatment to cure cancers. When these alternatives are not available, screening may be applicable if, and only if, it has been shown to reduce mortality from the disease.

Preventing cancer through primary care

Primary care teams are exceptionally well placed to provide a focus for cancer prevention and early diagnosis for the following reasons.

1. Coverage—primary care provides access to almost the entire population.
2. Health promotion and screening—in accordance with the 1990 general practitioner contract (see the Appendix), primary care now encompasses a comprehensive process of health promotion and screening.
3. Practice registers—these provide an ideal (if at present inaccurate) basis for the provision of cancer screening.
4. Advice—lifestyle advice given in general practice can be effective (e.g. advice to stop smoking).
5. Motivation—primary care can provide a source of encouragement for the less motivated and those who do not attend for screening.
6. Continuum of care—general practice offers a continuum of care which is important because any preventive intervention should be followed through on a long-term basis.

The potential contribution of primary care to cancer control can be summarized as follows.

- Prevention—facilitate changes in lifestyle, increase awareness of risk and what (if anything) can be done to reduce it.
- Early diagnosis—increase awareness of the potential benefits of early diagnosis, help individuals by understanding the attitudes and beliefs which influence decision making.

The key ways in which primary care can help are summarized in Box 16.1. Any intervention planned through primary care, particularly in terms of effecting lifestyle changes, should be integrated into more general programmes concerned with chronic disease prevention. As a result this chapter links with those on cardiovascular disease, smoking, diet, and alcohol. For this reason we have dealt only briefly with lifestyle issues in this chapter, concentrating primarily on breast and cervical screening.

Box 16.1: The role of the primary care team in cancer control

Advising people how to stop smoking.
Preventing alcohol misuse.
Giving appropriate dietary advice.
Advising people to avoid excessive exposure to sunshine.
Identifying and advising eligible women about breast cancer screening.
Running an effective cervical cytology programme.

It should be noted that any contribution by the health services has to be complemented by action taken in other spheres, most notably political action to reduce the prevalence of smoking.

Social class and cancer

With the exception of breast cancer and melanoma, cancer incidence rates for all other cancers are higher in social classes 4 and 5 than in social classes 1 and 2. The reasons for this are complex and varied. A few points should be emphasized which primary care teams will need to bear in mind when planning their cancer control strategy.

1. There is no evidence that those in social classes 4 and 5 are less concerned about cancer than those in social classes 1 and 2.
2. Those in social class 4 and 5 may be preoccupied with problems other than cancer risk reduction such as poverty, bad housing, and unemployment. Nonetheless they have the right to be informed about health options and to be given appropriate support.
3. In general people from social classes 4 and 5 make less use of preventive services, in part because health is a lower priority, in part because the services tend to be more attuned to the expectations and wishes of those in social classes 1 and 2. Thus, for example, cervical screening has failed to reach those at relatively higher risk of developing the disease, namely older women of lower social classes.
4. The pattern of cancer mortality in women is changing, with lung cancer beginning to overtake breast cancer as the leading cause of female cancer deaths (this has already occurred in Scotland). There is a strong reverse trend between smoking and social class, the prevalence being much higher in social classes 4 and 5.

Lifestyle changes

Smoking

This is the single most important cause of cancer, being significantly more important than all the others. In total approximately 30 per cent of all cancer deaths are attributable to tobacco smoking, that is most lung cancer deaths and a proportion of deaths from cancers of the mouth, pharynx, larynx, oesophagus, bladder, probably the pancreas, and possibly the kidney and cervix (see Table 16.1). Four points summarize the risk of lung cancer from smoking (see Box 16.2). GPs and practice nurses have a key role in helping patients to stop smoking. This is dealt with in detail in Chapter 9.

Alcohol

Second only in importance to smoking as a proven cause of cancer is alcohol (see Table 16.2). In conjunction with tobacco it may be responsible for as

Table 16.1 Cancer deaths due to smoking (USA, 1985). (Source: Surgeon General 1989)

Type of cancer	Per cent of deaths attributable to smoking	
	Men	Women
Lung	90	79
Lip, oral cavity, pharynx	92	61
Oesophagus	78	75
Bladder	47	37
Kidney	48	12
Larynx	81	87

Table 16.2 Cancers produced by alcohol consumption. (Source: Doll 1989)

	Cancers
Certainly produced	Mouth Pharynx Oesophagus Larynx Liver
Possibly produced	Breast Rectum

many as 10 per cent of all cancer deaths. The role of primary care teams in helping to reduce or cease alcohol consumption is described in Chapter 11.

Diet

The evidence on diet is as yet inconclusive. There is, however, accumulating data indicating that modifications in the diet may reduce the risk of cancer by as much as one-third. Practicable interventions which might reduce the risk of cancer are shown in Box 16.3. For several of these, however, the evidence is theoretical or contradictory and too weak to justify specific intervention. Any practical recommendations relating to alterations in the diet will need to be integrated with more general advice concerning diet and chronic disease prevention, rather than focusing specifically on the possible effects in reducing the risk of cancer. The subject of diet is covered in Chapter 10.

Box 16.2: Risk of lung cancer from smoking (Source: CRC 1989*a*)

Four points summarize the risk of lung cancer from smoking:

- Risk is directly related to the number of cigarettes* smoked, i.e. the higher the consumption, the higher the risk.
- Risk is more dependent on duration of smoking than on consumption, e.g. smoking one packet of cigarettes a day for 40 years is *eight times more hazardous* than smoking two packets a day for 20 years.
- Risk is reduced by ceasing to smoke. After ten or more years of giving up smoking, an ex-smoker has nearly the same risk as a non-smoker.
- Lower tar cigarettes appear to carry a lower risk of lung cancer than higher tar cigarettes.

* Smoking cigarettes carries a much higher risk than smoking other forms of tobacco.

Exposure to ultraviolet light

Exposure to the sun's ultraviolet rays can increase the risk of malignant melanoma. Malignant melanoma is a comparatively rare but serious form of skin cancer. There are currently 3100 new cases of malignant melanoma in the UK and 1200 deaths. Over the past decade there has been a dramatic increase in the number of people developing and dying from the disease in the UK. Moreover it is one of the few cancers to have a significant impact on young adults. 22 per cent of all malignant melanomas occur in the under 40s; in the age group 15 to 34 it is the fourth commonest cancer in women and the seventh commonest cancer in men.

Risk of malignant melanoma: prospects for prevention Several factors affect an individual's risk of malignant melanoma including some rare inherited characteristics (see Table 16.3). However, for the average individual three factors are important in predicting the risk of malignant melanoma: skin type, exposure to the sun, and changes in an existing mole.

Six skin types have been identified according to the ability of the skin to tan (see Table 16.4). people with skin types 1 and 2 are at greater risk of developing malignant melanoma whereas people with brown or black skin have a very low risk as their skin provides natural protection against the sun. The latest research confirms that if a person's skin has large numbers of naevi, both normal and atypical, and a tendency to freckle, then they are at a higher risk of developing malignant melanoma.

Exposure to the sun is the main aetiological factor linked with melanoma. Individuals with fair skin need high protection from the sun and it should be

Box 16.3: Dietary measures for the prevention of cancer (Doll 1989)

Measure	Type of cancer affected
• *Reduce intake*	
Calories (to avoid obesity)	Gall bladder Body of uterus Possibly breast
Fat	Breast Possibly colon, rectum
Smoked and grilled food	Stomach
Salt-cured food	Stomach
Nitrates	Stomach
Saccharin	Bladder
• *Increase consumption*	
Fibre and resistant starch	Colon, rectum
Green vegetables	Colon, rectum
Fruit	Stomach Possibly oesophagus
Vitamins A, C, E	Many sites
Beta-carotene	Many sites
Selenium	Many sites

Table 16.3 Individual risk factors for melanoma (CRC 1989*b*)

Risk factor and associated characteristics	Relative risk
Hair colour blonde or red	3
Skin colour: type 1 or 2. Poor tanning ability	3
History of severe sunburn	3
Previous primary melanoma. Risk of second primary	8
Large numbers of 'normal' naevi. Young people, over 100 naevi Large numbers of 'normal' naevi. Older people, over 50 naevi	20–30
Dysplastic naevi. No family history of melanoma	4–10
Dysplastic naevi. Family history of melanoma	100–400
Having a mole changing in shape or colour	400

Table 16.4 Skin types, sun exposure, and sunscreens (CRC 1989*b*)

Skin type	Sun screen (SPF number)
1. White skin, never tans, always burns	15 or higher in strong light at all times
2. White skin, burns initially, tans with difficulty 3. White skin, tans easily, burns rarely 4. White skin, never burns, always tans Mediterranean type	8–15 according to sunlight intensity
5. Brown skin 6. Black skin	Rarely need a sunscreen

noted that children are at risk of developing malignant melanoma later in life if overexposed to the sun in infancy.

Unlike skin type which a person cannot change, exposure to the sun is a risk factor that can be modified provided that the individual is aware of the dangers.

GPs and practice nurses have an increasingly important role to play, both in providing accurate information for their patients about primary melanoma prevention and in facilitating early diagnosis of melanoma. They can provide practical advice to those most at risk, either opportunistically or in the context of well-person clinics. Some guidelines for risk reduction are shown in Box 16.4.

Changes in an existing mole: encouraging skin surveillance and early reporting Survival of patients treated when their melanoma is at an early stage of its development before it has metastasized, is very good. Prognosis is

Box 16.4: Guidelines for risk reduction of malignant melanoma

- Ration exposure to strong sunlight.
- Keep out of the strong midday sun.
- Use a sunscreen (to shield from UVB light) or a sunblock (to shield from UVA and UVB light) as appropriate—see Table 16.4.
- Protect children and infants from strong sunlight at all times. Use a high-SPF sunscreen (SPF 15+).
- Remember clothing is a most effective sunscreen.
- Avoid the use of sunbeds.

directly related to the thickness of the tumour, known as the Breslow thickness. Patients with 'thin' tumours at the time of surgery have very high survival.

To help people evaluate the importance of changes in an existing mole, a seven-point checklist has been devised (Mackie 1989). People are advised to visit a doctor if an existing mole changes in size, shape, or colour or if three of the following four features are seen: diameter is 7 mm or greater; inflammation; oozing, crusting or bleeding; and itchiness.

Changes in size, shape (asymmetry and an irregular outline), and colour (irregular—a variety of shades of brown and black) warrant immediate referral. The additional presence of one or more of the four other features adds to the possibility that the diagnosis is melanoma, but on their own they do not in general warrant referral.

Early detection

Introduction

The purpose of screening for early detection of cancer is to interrupt the natural history of development of the cancer, and thereby to prevent it from progressing to a more advanced stage and ultimately death. Screening is not the first choice in any cancer control programme because:

1. it implies subjecting large numbers of healthy individuals to a medical procedure which, for the vast majority, will not do any good and may cause some harm;
2. the growth rates of most cancers are variable and it is unlikely that screening can influence all cases favourably.
3. many of the very early abnormalities detected by screening may not necessarily have progressed, i.e. overdiagnosis may occur.

Screening should thus only be considered when primary prevention or effective treatment are not feasible alternatives. Because of the problems outlined above, the evidence for any screening procedure needs to be rigorously evaluated against clear criteria, a proven benefit must be demonstrated in terms of a mortality reduction, and a careful balance must be struck between the benefits and the costs.

Weighing up the benefits and adverse effects

The benefits and disadvantages of screening are summarized in Chapter 8. The following points in particular should be noted.

1. Screening tests have, like almost all diagnostic tests, limitations. They do not detect 100 per cent of people with the disease or precursor condition (giving rise to false negatives) and they label some people as positive who do not actually have the disease (giving rise to false positives). The degree

to which a test diagnoses the condition sought is called the sensitivity, and the degree to which the test is able to correctly identify those who do not have the disease is called the specificity.

2. The limitations of any screening test must be made clear to those being offered the test, for example by the use of appropriate health education material.
3. Screening has adverse effects. Those who are in fact false positives may suffer unnecessary anxiety and may be subjected to further tests or investigations which may themselves carry a morbidity. Furthermore, not all those diagnosed correctly as having the disease will benefit from the diagnosis. For example, in breast cancer screening the programme will identify about 90 per cent of the cancers in the women who actually present for screening but the reduction in mortality in this group will only be about 40 per cent. Thus for more than half of those who have a cancer detected there will be no reduction in mortality, but an increased period knowing of the presence of the disease.
4. At first sight it might seem that early detection will always improve prognosis, but the longer survival of people diagnosed with an earlier stage of cancer might in fact be explicable solely because of the earlier diagnosis itself, with the mortality from the disease not reduced. The sole effect in these circumstances is that the individual knows that he or she has cancer for a longer period of time.

   This is called lead-time basis. It represents a major problem in assessing early diagnosis of cancer. In consequence it is necessary to demonstrate a reduction in mortality using a randomized controlled trial. In this way bias is eliminated and survival can be compared in those who have been offered a screening test with those who have not, before any decision can be reached about the efficacy of a screening test.
5. Many of the psychological problems resulting from false positive tests can be prevented or at least minimized by the provision of adequate counselling and support, and by ensuring rapid follow-up after the initial test. No health service should introduce screening without adequate resources for investigation, follow-up, and counselling and support.
6. A screening test, for example, mammography or the cervical smear test, should never itself be considered as being synonymous with screening. The term 'screening' should be used to refer to all those tests and investigations which are required in order to establish a diagnosis. Screening tests should only be offered in the context of well organized screening programmes aimed at defined populations.

Bearing in mind the points made above, screening for the following cancers will be discussed.

- breast
- cervix

- colorectal
- ovarian
- testicular.

Early detection of melanoma was covered previously in this chapter.

Cancer screening is as yet of proven value for only two cancer sites—breast and cervix. For this reason most of the following discussion will concentrate on these two cancers.

Breast cancer screening

Introduction

Each year there are over 26 000 new cases of breast cancer in the UK and nearly 16 000 deaths. There are at present no prospects for primary prevention and there are as yet only moderate improvements in the treatment of the disease.

Breast cancer screening provides an important alternative strategy. It is designed to detect invasive breast cancer at a very early stage, or to detect ductal carcinoma *in situ*. Its efficacy in reducing mortality from breast cancer in women aged 50 years and over has been demonstrated in randomized controlled studies. On the basis of the evidence, the authors of the *Forrest Report*, published in 1986, concluded that there was a convincing case on clinical grounds to provide mammographic screening on a UK basis. A national screening programme was accordingly set up from March 1988 and is currently being phased in.

The NHS breast screening programme provides an important new challenge to the whole primary care team. The programme follows the recommendations made in the *Forrest Report*: women aged 50–64 years will be invited for mammography, women aged 65 years and over will have mammography on request; women under 50 years will not be offered routine mammography. Single oblique-view mammography is to take place at three-yearly intervals. These guidelines are being kept under review and are the subject of national research trials.

The success of any screening programme depends on high participation of the target population, and a high-quality service. If 70 per cent of the invited population attend for breast screening of high quality, the reduction in mortality should result in the prevention of about 1200 deaths each year in women in this age group, although the full effect of the screening programme will not be observed until about the year 2000.

The screening procedure

The screening procedure can be divided into three stages:

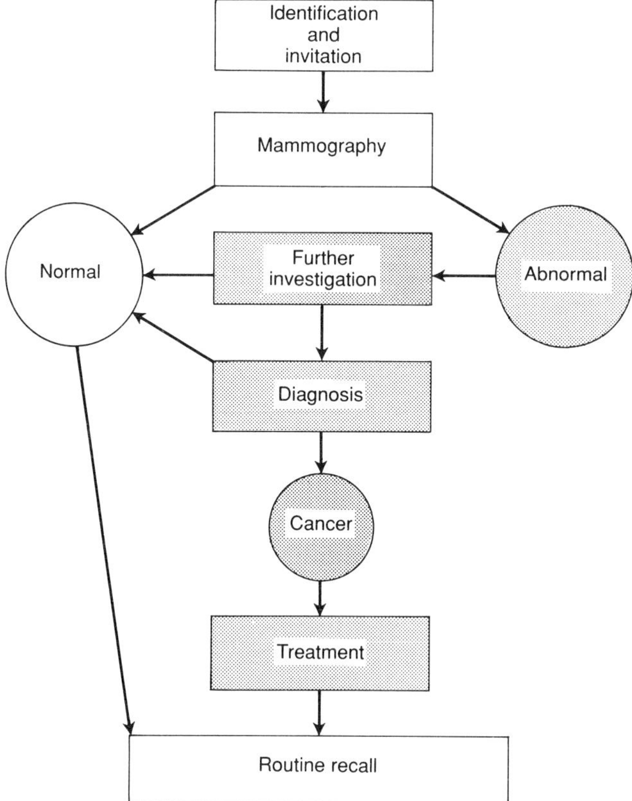

Fig. 16.4 The breast screening procedure.

1. identification and invitation;
2. mammography;
3. further investigation, followed by treatment.

The relationship between these stages is shown in Fig. 16.4.

Mammography is carried out at a basic screening unit which can be mobile or static. Further investigation of mammographically detected abnormalities is carried out at specially established assessment centres. These should have multidisciplinary teams with the necessary skills, experience, and equipment to localize, excise, and examine impalpable lesions and ensure that the number of recalls and invasive procedures are kept to a minimum.

The numbers of women involved at each stage of the screening procedure are shown in Fig. 16.5.

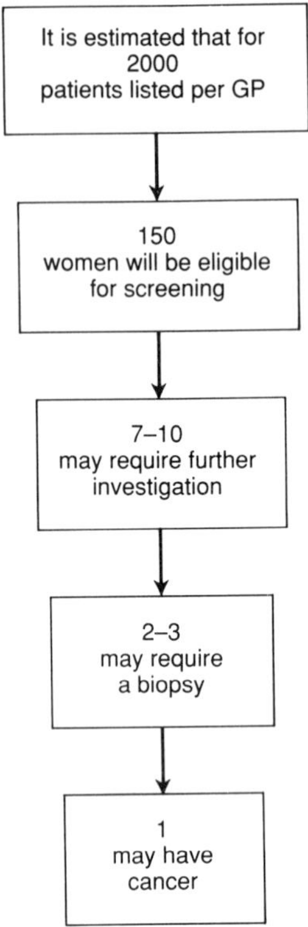

Fig. 16.5 Numbers of women at each stage of breast screening (assuming 100% acceptance).

The role of the primary care team

Because it was recognized as being necessary to concentrate the skills required for further investigation, most screening programmes cover more than one District Health Authority. Standard practice is for the screening programme to work with one primary care team at a time, moving steadily round the population to be covered. Because of the importance attached to the part that primary care teams can play, the local screening office will make contact with primary care teams some months before their population is actually due to be covered. It is standard practice for a visit to be made to the primary care team to discuss its involvement in the programme.

Primary care teams can help to improve the quality of the programme, increase uptake, and provide information and advice by carrying out the tasks listed in Box 16.5. Experience has shown that the workload implica-

Box 16.5: Breast screening: the practical contribution of the primary care team

Quality
- Improve acceptability of the programme.
- Make appropriate referral arrangements.
- Evaluate primary care involvement.

Uptake
- Check Prior Notification Lists (PNLs).
- Encourage attendance.
- Provide practical advice.
- Allay fears.
- Discuss screening with non-attenders.

Information and counselling
- Answer general enquiries.
- Advise ineligible women.
- Discuss the implications of recall for further investigation.
- Discuss the implications of a biopsy.
- Discuss treatment options.
- Discuss screening with non-attenders.

tions for primary care teams are not excessive. Guidelines relating to the management of specific categories of women are given in Box 16.6.

Counselling women recalled for further investigation

An abnormal result will create anxiety, and general practitioners can help in allaying fears, although most often in the breast screening programme these fears and anxieties are dealt with by the staff at the assessment centre. Women may wish their general practitioners to provide information about the implications of a result that requires further investigation. It is important therefore to appreciate the complexity and limitations of mammography and the corresponding need to call back a number of women who will subsequently be found to be normal. It is equally important, however, not to provide false reassurance at this stage. General practitioners will need to be able to explain the range of diagnostic techniques that are available and what these may entail. Most women who have abnormal mammograms will be found to be normal on assessment and will rejoin the routine recall system. Some women will have cancer diagnosed by fine-needle aspiration cytology and will not need a biopsy. A few may require a biopsy to allow a firm diagnosis or exclude the possibility of cancer.

Box 16.6: Guidelines for GPs about specific categories of women

- Women under 50: There is insufficient evidence to demonstrate that screening women under 50 is effective in reducing mortality from breast cancer. The risks may be greater than any potential benefit.
- Women with a family history of breast cancer: Women under 50 should not automatically be included in the screening programme solely on account of their family history. Women aged 50 and over with a family history should not be offered screening more frequently than once every three years unless there are mammographic or clinical indications for doing so.
- Women with symptoms between routine mammograms: Women should continue to be aware of minimal symptoms and report these without delay to their GPs even if they have been recently screened. A woman with symptoms should be examined by her GP and, if necessary, be referred for investigation as at present either to a hospital breast clinic or to a general surgical outpatients clinic.
- Women with breast cancer: Women aged 50 and over with breast cancer should remain on the call/recall system, and continue to have mammograms at least every three years on the other breast and, in the case of breast conservation, on the treated breast.
- Women on hormone replacement therapy (HRT): Women aged 50 to 64 who are receiving HRT do not need to have more frequent screening. Women do not require a baseline mammogram before receiving HRT.

Non-attenders

If a woman does not attend for mammography her general practitioner will be informed. This information should be recorded in her notes, preferably with an external marker for easy identification. General practitioners, practice nurses, and health visitors are in an ideal position to discuss breast screening with non-attenders, either when the woman next consults or directly by contacting non-attenders to offer further information and advice. If the woman has fears and anxieties these need to be carefully explored. Remember that ultimately women have the right to choose not to participate in the screening programme. They should have access to accurate information to enable them to arrive at an informed decision. It is important not to create feelings of guilt or inadequacy by this process.

Cervical cancer screening

Background

At present the exact cause of cervical cancer is not known, so primary prevention is not feasible. Cervical cancer screening or secondary prevention can, however, prevent an invasive cancer developing in that it aims in particular to identify cervical intraepithelial neoplasia, the pre-invasive stage of cervical cancer.

Because cervical screening started before the era of randomized controlled trials, there are no such trials demonstrating its effeciveness in reducing mortality. The evidence for its benefit is derived mainly from the comparison of trends in mortality in those countries in which there is well organized screening and those countries which in the past have not had well organized screening, the United Kingdom falling into the latter category. Nearly complete coverage of the target population by organized cervical screening programmes in Iceland, Finland, Sweden, and parts of Denmark were soon followed by sharp falls in both incidence and mortality. In the UK on the other hand there has been considerable variation in the age-specific mortality trends, as shown in Fig. 16.6. However, any observed increase in mortality may well have been greater in the absence of screening:

Risk factors

The risk of developing cervical cancer is closely related to sexual habits, with very low rates of the disease in nuns. Early age at first intercourse and multiple partners (often these two factors go together) are high risk factors, and the risk for a woman is raised with the number of sexual contacts her partner has had.

The causes of the disease are not known but a sexually transmitted infection (possibly genital wart virus) is implicated, although this has not been proved with any degree of certainty. In general, women of low socio-economic status have higher rates of the disease and women in developing countries are at greater risk than women in the developed world. Smoking is thought to increase a woman's susceptibility to the disease and a history of dysplasia increases a woman's risk of developing invasive carcinoma.

The scope for secondary prevention

About 4500 women develop cervical cancer each year and just over 2000 die from it. The statement is sometimes made that there are '2000 avoidable deaths'. There is, however, little evidence that all these deaths are 'avoidable'.

The fact that the total number of deaths has remained fairly constant over several decades not only hides the fact that mortality rates are decreasing in

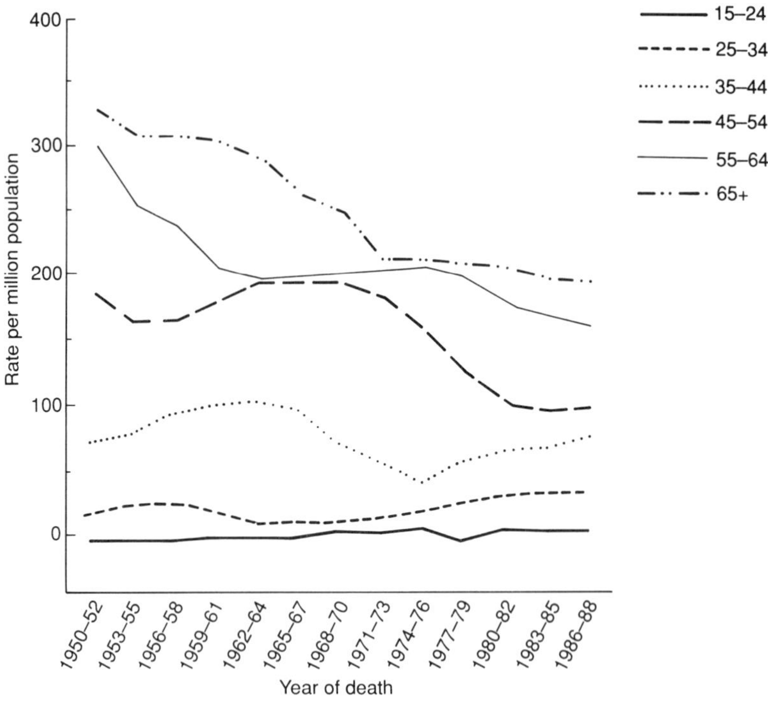

Fig. 16.6 Invasive carcinoma of the cervix uteri: mortality rates by age, England and Wales 1950–88. (From CRC 1990)

certain age groups (see Fig. 16.6), but also that the programme may indeed have been effective in preventing a rise in mortality from cervical cancer, because it does appear that the precursor condition, cervical intraepithelial neoplasia, is increasing in incidence, although the natural history of the disease is not fully understood.

The precise proportion of the 2000 deaths that are preventable is not easy to calculate but as many as one-third or one-half may well be preventable by early detection and the prompt treatment of neoplastic and pre-neoplastic lesions.

The NHS cervical cancer screening programme

Until recently the cervical cancer screening programme in the UK has had a chaotic history. The introduction in 1988 of a systematic call and recall system and the setting up of an NHS Cervical Screening Programme National Co-ordinating Network has brought a greater sense of coherence. Steps have been taken by District and Regional Health Authorities nationally to improve the effectiveness of the cervical screening programme.

The role of the primary care team

Primary care teams have a key role in ensuring the success of cervical screening, contributing to it in several fundamental ways. The contribution of primary care teams is summarized in Box 16.7 and guidelines are shown in Box 16.8.

Box 16.7: Cervical screening: primary care activities

Setting up and running a systematic screening programme.
Improving coverage of the target population.
Following up women who did not respond to the invitation.
Taking cervical smears.
Communicating with the laboratory.
Dealing with normal smear results.
Dealing with 'not normal' smear results.
Reducing patient anxiety and dissatisfaction.
Running an effective fail-safe system.
Evaluating the screening programme.

Box 16.8: Guidelines for cervical screening

- Who should be screened? All women aged 20 to 64 who are or ever have been sexually active.
- How often should smears be taken? At least every five years.
- Which women need more frequent smears? Women who have had an abnormal smear, or have been treated for CIN lesions and for squamous carcinomas, may require more frequent smears (see Table 16.5).

Although there are several risk factors associated with an increased risk of invasive carcinoma of the cervix, these factors cannot be used to predict reliably which women will develop CIN. There is thus little value in selecting these women for more frequent screening.

Although cell changes suggesting infection with wart virus (HPV) are no longer in themselves considered an indication for more frequent screening, the majority of smears showing evidence of HPV will also have nuclear abnormalities described as 'dyskaryosis' or 'borderline' and should be managed accordingly (see Table 16.5).

Taking the smear

The basic screening test is the cervical smear test. The objective of the test is to identify women whose cytological pattern is suggestive of CIN. One of the key factors determining the effectiveness of a cervical screening programme is the quality of smear taking. Poor smear taking can miss 20 per cent or more of pre-cancerous abnormalities in the cervix.

The smear itself is taken by scraping cells from the cervix at the junction between the endocervix (covered by columnar epithelium) and the ectocervix (covered by squamous epithelium). The anatomical position of the transformation zone varies. It is thought that the initial changes in carcinogenesis take place here and therefore it is important to get cells from both the endo- and ectocervix.

Primary screening should be carried out with an Aylesbury spatula which has a tip that is longer than the Ayres spatula and is thought to be more likely to sample endocervical cells as well as transformation zone squamous cells The flatter reverse end may be used for a patulous cervix or a vault smear.

A cytobrush is used to sample the endocervix and is mainly used in colposcopy clinics or when the cervix is distorted by surgery or local ablation. It may be used in addition to a spatula in some instances. It is not the method of choice in primary screening because it does not always sample the transformation zone and provides smears of sparse cellularity which dry quickly and need very rapid fixation.

A cervical smear if properly taken should contain cells from the whole of the transformation zone which should therefore be adequately sampled. Squamous epithelial cells will normally be the most numerous cell type. The main evidence of an adequate smear is that it should contain a sufficient quantity of epithelial cells, taking into account a woman's age and her hormonal status.

An indication that the transformation zone has been properly sampled is the additional presence of endocervical columnar cells and recognizable metaplastic cells. Due to the variable nature of the transformation zone only one of these cell types may be present on the smear. Endocervical cells may not always be seen in smears from post-menopausal women or those with atrophic smears.

Taking adequate smears will remove the anxiety for those women asked to return for repeat smears and reduce the overall workload for practices. Also, in the terms of the GP contract, the calculation of targets are based on adequate smear tests only.

The appearance that is noted when cells are scraped from the surface of CIN lesions is called 'dyskaryosis'. Cytological reports of dyskaryosis are usually classified as mild, moderate, or severe.

The screening test is about 80 per cent sensitive, with a specificity of the same order. However, sensitivity and specificity are difficult to calculate from routine cervical screening data.

Interpretation of the smear results

Smear results can sometimes be difficult to interpret. The smear may be normal in that there is no significant nuclear abnormality, but other comments may also be made about the smear. When a smear is reported with some abnormal cells, the action required will depend on many factors including the appearance of any previous smears.

Smears should be coded as 'negative' if there is no nuclear abnormality, in which case a repeat smear will *not* be necessary unless there is a history of previous abnormal smears or CIN.

All abnormal cervical smears should be assigned a result code depending on the degree of nuclear abnormality, as an indicator of neoplasia or intra-epithelial neoplasia (see Table 16.5).

HPV infection is suggested by koilocytosis, individual cell keratinization, and binucleation, and is most often associated with nuclear changes indistinguishable from mild dyskaryosis. Such smears should be coded according to the degree of nuclear change and managed according to the predicted grade of CIN and not simply the presence of HPV. Changes suggesting HPV infection *without* nuclear changes are rare. These should be coded 'negative' and will not, therefore, indicate the need for more frequent follow-up. The presence of a viral change should *not* be recorded if it will not alter the management of the woman (i.e. it is not accompanied by nuclear changes).

There is currently no justification for managing mild dyskaryosis by colposcopy. One borderline or mildly dyskaryotic smear should be managed by a repeat smear at six months and consideration given to colposcopic referral if still not normal. A minimum of two consecutive negative smears are needed before return to normal screening frequency.

Other terminology may be used in describing smears which are negative. In some cases these may require other action by the GP, e.g. in the case of specific infections such as *Candida*- or *Actinomyces*-like organisms. As long as there is no nuclear abnormality a repeat smear will not be necessary. Routine recall should be recommended.

Who needs colposcopy

Moderate and severe dyskaryosis should be an indication for colposcopy. A borderline or mildly dyskaryotic smear should be managed by a repeat smear at six months with referral for colposcopy only if the abnormality persists. Referrals for colposcopy should be based on the degree of dyskaryosis with the exception of the clinically suspicious cervix which should indicate referral to a gynaecologist for appropriate investigation and biopsy regardless of the smear result.

Table 16.5 Interpretation of smear results. (Note: The term 'atypical cells' is no longer recommended in the Result Codes and its use should be discontinued. The preferred term is 'borderline changes'.) (Source: BSCC 1989, Duncan 1991)

Result code	Explanation	Action
Inadequate	Insufficient cellular material Inadequate fixation Smear consisting mainly of blood or inflammatory cell exudate Little or no material to suggest that the transformation zone has been sampled	Repeat smear
Negative	Normal. Includes simple inflammatory changes including a mild polymorph exudate	Routine recall
Borderline changes, with or without HPV change	Cellular appearances that cannot be described as normal. Smears in which there is doubt as to whether the nuclear changes are inflammatory or dyskaryosis	Repeat smear at six months. Consider for colposcopy if changes persist
Mild dyskaryosis with or without HPV change	Cellular appearances consistent with origin from CIN 1 (mild dysplasia)	Repeat smear at six months. Consider for colposcopy if changes persist
Moderate dyskaryosis with or without HPV change	Cellular appearances consistent with origin from CIN 2 (moderate dysplasia)	Refer for colposcopy
Severe dyskaryosis with or without HPV change	Cellular appearances consistent with origin from CIN 3 (severe dysplasia/carcinoma in situ)	Refer for colposcopy
Severe dyskaryosis / ? invasive carcinoma	Cellular appearances consistent with origin from CIN 3, but with additional features which suggest the possibility of invasive cancer	Refer for colposcopy
Glandular neoplasia or suspicion of glandular neoplasia	Cellular appearances suggesting pre-cancer or cancer in the cervical canal or the endometrum	Refer for colposcopy

At colposcopy samples can be taken from the cervix using a punch biopsy and if histological diagnosis indicates CIN 2 or 3, the affected part of the cervix is removed or destroyed. In the past this was always done by cone biopsy under general anaesthetic but increasing use is now made of a large cutting electrosurgical loop which can remove the affected part of the cervix and the whole of the transformation zone where the squamous epithelium of the vaginal covering of the cervix becomes transformed into the columnar epithelium of the cervical canal itself. Women with CIN 1 may be treated or kept under close surveillance.

Colposcopy itself should not be painful for the patient, but can be uncomfortable and requires her to be prone with her feet in stirrups or knees held up and apart over supports. Large loop excision or diathermy may be painful in some instances and there may be an unpleasant smell and some bleeding. Patients should be carefully prepared for these procedures.

Giving results

It is important to ensure that results are effectively communicated to women. Results should be conveyed *in writing* whether the result is normal or abnormal. The way in which a patient is told about an abnormal smear will often affect how she will cope with any treatment or future follow-up. According to recent research, information and support are needed particularly in the following areas, to avoid unnecessary anxiety:

- Informing women of the result: It is essential to ensure that the information is understandable and not alarming. Women who need a referral to colposcopy or who have invasive disease should be offered an early appointment or opportunity to speak with the GP to discuss the implications of the results. Waiting and uncertainty are often the most difficult part of the referral process.
- Explaining the meaning of an abnormal result: If the result is not normal it is often assumed that it means cancer. It is therefore important to explain exactly what the abnormality is, what it may be due to, and what further steps in investigation, follow-up, and treatment are needed. Explaining terms, e.g. dyskaryosis, CIN, and preinvasive cancer, is important.
- Explaining investigation and treatment: Many women do not know what will be involved when they are referred for colposcopy and therefore this needs explanation. Also explain possible treatments such as cone biopsy, laser treatment, or hysterectomy, before a woman is referred. Depending on age, many will want to know how the treatment will affect their sex lives and their chances of future pregnancies.
- Giving practical advice: Give information about intercourse, future contraception, pregnancy, and the use of tampons, as patients may feel inhibited about discussing these issues.

- Arranging future follow-up: Always consider inviting the patient for future follow-up by the GP after she has attended the hospital, as this can be very reassuring.

Follow-up of treated patients

Cytological follow-up is essential after treatment for CIN. Colposcopy is not essential but may enhance detection of persistent disease. There are four reasons for follow-up.

1. To identify residual disease.
2. To identify new CIN.
3. To identify new invasive disease.
4. To reassure both the patient and the clinician.

There is no evidence to support the continuing use of colposcopy in the review process. Those patients who have undergone ablation or excision should be followed up cytologically. An endocervical brush may be needed if the cervix has healed with a very small aperture.

In patients with conservatively treated CIN 3, increased surveillance need not be continued beyond five years. A first cytological review should be undertaken at six months, and then, if normal, be repeated at 12 months. Patients should then be returned to the GP for yearly follow up and at five years returned to the normal screening frequency. A normal smear at six months does not warrant further colposcopic assessment.

Post-hysterectomy the risks of residual or new disease are very low provided that the woman was colposcopically assessed prior to surgery to exclude occult disease at the top of the vagina. Women who have had a hysterectomy for benign disease need not be kept under routine surveillance. Women who have had a hysterectomy for pre-malignancy should have persistent disease excluded by cytology at six months and one year after surgery and then no further smears if the cytology is normal.

The psychological effects of cervical screening

There is no firm evidence that either the herpes or the papilloma viruses cause or precipitate cervical cancer. Nevertheless there is a widespread belief among the public and among professionals that cervical cancer is in some ways a sexually transmitted disease. A report of 'infection' may come as a considerable shock to many people and depression, guilt, and marital and sexual problems can result.

If the woman is told that she has CIN there is obviously concern about the possibility of cancer. There is considerable confusion about the difference between intraepithelial neoplasia and invasive neoplasia. In addition the connotation of infection and sexually transmitted disease can further aggravate the adverse psychological impact of diagnosis.

These problems are severe enough if the woman actually has CIN, but if referral for colposcopy is made and the woman does not turn out to have CIN, the adverse psychological sequelae will have been incurred without benefit to the woman. A certain proportion of false positives are inevitable, as in any screening test, and the challenge is therefore to minimize the number of false positives and to minimize the proportion of women referred for colposcopy.

The psychological impact of the diagnosis of infection or CIN, or the referral for colposcopy can be minimized by:

1. The provision of clear written information at all stages of the screening process.
2. The availability of a phone number and the possibility to discuss the problem with a sympathetic person.
3. The provision of counselling by the person carrying out colposcopy.
4. A reduction in delays in reporting and in waiting for colposcopy if needed.

Screening for other cancers

Colorectal cancer

This is one of the commonest cancers in the UK, but mortality rates have remained more or less constant over the past few decades. Screening is a very attractive proposition because of the very great difference in prognosis between early (Dukes' stage A) cases and the later stages where infiltration through the bowel wall has already occurred. Moreover, it is thought that large polypoid adenomas of the colon and rectum are in many cases precursors of malignant change. Their identification and removal might reduce the subsequent incidence of invasive cancer. Screening might result, therefore, in lowered incidence and mortality. A number of tests for faecal occult blood have been developed and these provide a cheap and easy method of screening although not always acceptable to the population (Chamberlain 1988).

Randomized controlled studies of faecal occult blood screening are currently in progress in the US, Sweden, Denmark, and Nottingham in the UK. None has so far shown a mortality reduction. Until at least the trial in Nottingham reports in 1995, there is no case for providing colorectal screening as a service.

Ovarian cancer

Ovarian cancer affects just over 5000 women a year. The prognosis is poor with only a 28 per cent five-year relative survival rate and over 4200 deaths a year.

Screening for ovarian cancer by ultrasound, or by serum levels of a monoclonal antibody, CA 125, has shown that it is possible to detect ovarian cancer at an early stage, although at the price of a large number of false positive results. A feasibility study for a randomized controlled trial is currently in progress in the UK. Until such time as its efficacy in reducing deaths from this disease is proven, screening for ovarian cancer should not, in the light of current knowledge, be offered as a routine test.

Testicular cancer

Testicular cancer is the commonest cause of cancer among young men in the UK accounting for 16 per cent of all male cancers at ages 20–44. The majority of testicular cancer cases occur at ages 30–34. There has been a marked increase in incidence over the past 15 years. In contrast mortality rates have fallen. This fall is a consequence of the recent dramatic improvement in survival that has taken place due to major advances in treatment. At present 95 per cent of early stage tumours are curable.

Early diagnosis is crucial in improving prognosis. It is likely to be associated with simpler and less toxic treatment and more likely to be followed by cure.

More than 90 per cent of patients with testicular germ cell tumours present with a swelling of the testis. It is very rare for the patient not to be aware of the testicular abnormality and delay in diagnosis is not usually due to this cause. Rather delay reflects reluctance of the patient to consult the GP, sometimes out of fear or embarrassment, but often because of lack of awareness that a potentially serious and progressive illness may arise in the testis.

Delay in referral from general practice to hospital also occurs. This can be avoided by full understanding of the differential diagnosis of testicular tumours and epididymitis, or by the practice of reassessment of testicular abnormalities even if they are thought to be benign on initial assessment.

Although screening by routine self-examination has been proposed this is of unproven benefit. There are no firm data on the specificity of self-examination but, from anecdotal reports, its widespread application might lead to a substantial increase in investigation of nonmalignant conditions. There is, therefore, no case for providing testicular self-examination screening.

Summary

Primary care teams have an important part to play in both the prevention of cancer and its early detection.

In prevention the primary care team can play a part in helping to bring about changes in smoking behaviour, alcohol consumption, and diet, changes which will of course not only reduce the risk of cancers, but also the risk of other diseases, notably cardiovascular disease. Increasingly, in part because of growing public awareness, in part because of increasing risk, people will be turning to general practitioners for advice on reducing the risk of malignant melanoma.

In the early detection of asymptomatic cancer primary care teams play a centrally important part in breast and cervical cancer screening.

References and further reading

Austoker, J. (1990). *Breast cancer screening.* Meditext, London.

Austoker, J. and McPherson, A. (1992). *Cervical screening.* Oxford University Press, Oxford.

BSCC (1989). *Taking cervical smears*, p. 18. Aspen Corporate Communications, London.

Chamberlain (1988). Screening for early detection of cancer. In *Oncology for nurses and health care professionals*, Vol. 1, (ed. R. Tiffany and A. P. Pritchard), pp. 155–73. Harper and Row, London.

CRC (1989a). *Lung cancer and smoking*, Cancer Research Campaign Factsheet 11. CRC, London.

CRC (1989b). *Malignant melanoma*, Cancer Research Campaign Factsheet 4. CRC London.

CRC (1990). *Cancer of the cervix uteri*, Cancer Research Campaign Factsheet 12. CRC, London.

Doll, R. (1989). The prevention of cancer: opportunities and challenges. In *Reducing the risk of cancer* (ed. T. Heller, B. Davey, and L. Bailey), pp. 14–25. Hodder and Stoughton, London.

Doll, R. and Peto, R. (1981). *The causes of cancer.* Oxford University Press, Oxford.

Duncan, I. (ed.) (1991). *Draft guidelines for clinical practice and programme management.* NHS Cervical Screening Programme, Oxford.

Gray, M. (1991). *Breast cancer screening 1991: evidence and experience since the Forrest Report.* NHS BSP Publications, Sheffield.

Mackie, R. M. (1989). *Malignant melanoma: a guide to early diagnosis.* Glasgow.

Surgeon General (1989). Reducing the health consequences of smoking: 25 years of progress. Report of the Surgeon General, US Department of Health and Human Services, Maryland.

Vessey, M. P. and Gray, J. A. M. (ed.) (1986). *Cancer risks and cancer prevention.* Oxford University Press.

17 Communicable disease control

Richard Mayon-White

The communicable diseases present the most obvious and straightforward opportunities to practice preventive medicine, but include some of the most complex problems to control. New infectious diseases are being identified every year, mostly with alarming publicity. The outstanding problem of the last ten years is HIV/AIDS, which is dealt with in Chapter 18. In this chapter, the general principles are explained, because the general practitioner will have to use them to tackle unfamiliar problems. Within this chapter, the principles of communicable disease control are illustrated by focusing on particular diseases.

Surveillance

Surveillance of communicable diseases is a fundamental part of control. Surveillance is the various methods of finding and recording the incidence of disease, and making intelligent use of the information. Three methods are used in Britain:

1. Recording episodes of illness observed by general practitioners—sentinel practice schemes.
2. Regular reporting by laboratories to a central agency on microbiological diagnoses or epidemiological importance.
3. Notifications of infectious diseases to the 'proper officer' of the local authority.

Sentinel practices

Sentinel practice schemes were started by general practitioners for research and education, and have gained practical purposes from the continuity of records. With records on trends and patterns in disease, it is possible to respond responsibly to public fears about apparent increases in incidence. The records have special advantages because the population observed is clearly defined by the people registered with the GP, and the counts of cases are made as consistent as possible.

Surveillance uses epidemiological terms which should be defined.

Incidence is the number of new cases per unit of population in a set period of time, e.g. one case of pneumococcal pneumonia per 1000 people per year

Prevalence (often confused with incidence when used to say how common a disease is) is the number of cases (old and new) present in the population of unit size at a point in time. Prevalence is used for chronic diseases, but has its place in infections diseases for HIV infection and tuberculosis.

Two other words, outbreak and epidemic, cause confusion. In scientific language, the two words are synonymous, meaning a state in which a disease is occurring at a higher incidence than normal. Unfortunately the words are perceived to be alarming and have to be used cautiously in public statements. 'Outbreak' is used for events that seem to be limited in number and time, and 'epidemic' is reserved for larger, more extensive events. A typical outbreak is a cluster of cases occurring in one place in a short period of time with the suspicion that they have a single cause in common.

General Principles 1: Sentinel practice monitoring of the incidence of influenza

Influenza occurs in epidemics in most winters. It causes a marked increase in sickness absence from schools and work, and an increase in the number of deaths, for a period of three to four weeks. Sentinel practices detect these epidemics by a rise in the incidence of influenzal illness (upper respiratory symptoms with aching and fever) from 2 to 30 patients a week in a practice of 10 000 people. This tenfold rise is usually obvious within the practice, but it needs to be linked to what is happening elsewhere, particularly to laboratory isolates of influenza virus. The information is used to reassure the public and patients that the illness is influenza and to check that vaccines used in the previous autumn for people at high risk of complications had the correct composition. Doctors should no underestimate the reassurance gained from a confident statement on the diagnosis and size of an outbreak. Accurate information on the type of influenza virus and the age groups affected is used to decide the composition of vaccines in successive years.

Laboratory reports

Some countries have developed national surveillance systems based on laboratory records. In these, laboratories report regularly to a central agency on the number of diagnoses that they have made which may have epidemiological interest. In England, Wales, and Northern Ireland, these reports go to the Communicable Disease Surveillance Centre in London. The Communicable Diseases (Scotland) Unit in Glasgow is an older agency with the same function. These surveillance systems have the benefit of using proven diagnoses, but lack reliable denominators (size of population) to calculate incidence. The observed trends are mostly reliable, but can be affected by changes in access and attitudes to laboratory services.

General Principles 2: Laboratory monitoring of the incidence of cryptosporidiosis, and the importance of coordination

Cryptosporidiosis is a gastroenteritis which infects healthy people but is more severe and protracted in people with immunodeficiency. It may be water-borne or acquired from animal contact, although the majority of sporadic cases are in children who have been infected by their fellows. The water-borne outbreaks are the most important, and we rely on laboratories to detect them by a significant increase in the number of positive stool samples. Coordination between laboratories is necessary because water distribution areas are often larger than the catchment areas of laboratories. General practices are key services in the management of such an outbreak, as they are the primary source of diagnostic specimens and important routes of communication with those affected.

Notifications

Notification is the traditional method of surveillance, based on public health law. Those diseases that are notifiable are shown in Box 17.1. The system is due to be revised, to follow changes in the health services and modern knowledge of disease. At the time of writing, the notification is a paper form sent to the 'medical officer for environmental health', who is a doctor employed by a district health authority but holding an honorary post as a 'proper officer' of the local district or borough council. The legal powers to control notifiable diseases are held by the local council, not by the health authority. The powers include the exclusion of infected people from work or school, quarantine regulations, and compulsory medical examinations. One of the statutory duties related to notifiable diseases is the GP's or hospital clinician's duty to notify, for which a small fee is payable.

The duty to notify is often forgotten for diseases that do not present much threat to the public health (e.g. measles). The legal powers are rarely used,

Box 17.1: Notifiable diseases

Acute encephalitis
Acute poliomyelitis
Anthrax
Cholera
Diphtheria
Dysentery
Food poisoning
Leprosy
Leptospirosis
Malaria
Measles
Meningitis and meningococal septicaemia
Mumps
Ophthalmia neonatorum
Paratyphoid fever
Plague
Rabies
Relapsing fever
Rubella
Scarlet fever
Smallpox
Tetanus
Tuberculosis
Typhoid fever
Typhus
Viral haemorrhagic fever
Viral hepatitis
Whooping cough
Yellow fever

because most people can be persuaded to comply with sensible preventive measures. The emphasis on the formal aspects of notification is unfortunate, because it has delayed the modernization of this local surveillance system. 'Medical officers for environmental health' are being renamed as 'consultants for communicable disease control', officers of district health authorities. The actions that follow notification depend on the disease: whooping cough is recorded to monitor the immunization programme, so the information is only for statistical purposes. On the other hand, a report of typhoid fever raises questions and initiates actions by the public health department.

General Principles 3: The importance of the notification, and secondary prevention, of typhoid

Typhoid fever has become uncommon in Europe (about 100 cases in Britain each year). Nearly all cases are acquired by trvael to Africa or Asia. Primary prevention is by vaccination and advice on food hygiene for people travelling to these continents, including a reminder to those people who have emigrated from such countries that they also need protection. Typhoid is most commonly spread on food prepared by a carrier, who may or may not have had a clinical attack. Secondary prevention is advice to families of cases, exclusion of infected food-handlers from work, and the need to notify imported cases.

Investigation of outbreaks

By definition, outbreaks are events that are out of the usual. Once recognized, they require an explanation, and this often entails an investigation by the consultant for communicable disease control. Sometimes a GP can investigate an outbreak in a closed group, like a school where he or she is the medical officer. But there are advantages in getting the help of a specialist who can give an independent opinion, can use the resources of community nursing and environmental health departments, and can approach people who are registered with any medical practitioner. The steps taken to investigate outbreaks are not difficult, but are time-consuming (see Box 17.2).

Box 17.2: Investigation of outbreaks

1. Record all people who may have been affected, and decide who will be counted as a case.
2. Collect epidemiological histories and relevant specimens from the cases.
3. Work out to what the outbreak may be due.
4. Apply immediate control measures if known and feasible.
5. Test your theory with an analysis of the data, or by using an epidemiological method such as a case-control study.
6. Write a report that includes recommendations to prevent further outbreaks.
7. Follow up the investigation to check that your report was correct and was accepted.

General Principles 4: A population-based approach to outbreaks of food poisoning

Food poisoning is the commonest notifiable disease, although it is seriously under-reported, and it often occurs in outbreaks. Outbreaks should be reported as soon as possible in order to increase the chances of recovering the suspect food for laboratory tests, and to prevent further consumption of the food. There is no harm in reporting a suspected outbreak before there is laboratory confirmation of the clinical diagnosis (which could be elusive in a viral food-poisoning outbreak). Environmental health officers of the district council are the field force who take food histories, inspect premises, and arrange laboratory tests. They should, and normally do, involve the consultant for communicable disease control on the medical and epidemiological aspects of an outbreak of food poisoning. If the causative agent cannot be detected in food samples (often all the suspect food was consumed or thrown away immediately after the meal), much will depend on the quality of the epidemiology. If this is unconvincing, then caterers and consumers will not follow the advice to prevent further outbreaks.

Quarantine and isolation

Quarantine is one of the oldest methods of controlling infection, and it carries biblical and medieval images that can worry people who find themselves in an outbreak. The restrictions that were formerly imposed were irksome and were often circumvented. Applied selectively and sympathetically, some restictions have a worthy place in modern society: for example, quarantine for imported animals has prevented rabies entering Britain, with enormous benefits for people who care for animals or who are bitten by dogs, cats, or other mammals. Guidelines are shown in Box 17.3.

Box 17.3: Guidelines for quarantine and isolation

Rabies

- Notices on rabies precautions should be displayed in health cenres to warn overseas travellers not to bring animals back to Britain unless they use the quarantine kennels.

Fevers

- Patients with fevers should be nursed in single rooms until their diagnoses are established.
- Warn patients who may react to being isolated on admission.

Sonne dysentery

- Children should not go to school or nursery until their diarrhoea has settled.
- Explain this to parents, one of whom might have to stay at home from work for a few days.

Vaccination

Children

Vaccination is an effective means of controlling endemic infections like measles that spread from person to person, conditions in which isolation and quarantine fail. To be successful, a high uptake of vaccination is essential to from herd immunity. There will always be a few individuals who cannot be vaccinated because of hypersensitivity, immunodeficiency, or religious convictions. Their protection depends on reaching the other 99 per cent of the population. The main obstacle to high immunization rates is poor administration, not parental resistance. Efficient appointment systems, accurate patient registers, regular supplies of well-stored vaccine, and well-trained staff are the components of good administration. The new contractual arrangements that reward practices for high vaccination rates provide a useful incentive to those who are not protagonists of preventive medicine.

The new British schedule of vaccination is diphtheria/tetanus/pertussis (DTP) vaccine and oral polio at the ages of 2, 3, and 4 months of age. This is one of the youngest schedules in the world and still needs proof of efficacy. The triple DTP vaccine is likely to be joined by *Haemophilus influenzae* type b (Hib) vaccine as a national policy in October 1992. The diphtheria, tetanus, and polio vaccines need boosting, now at 4–5 years of age, and tetanus and polio are boosted again at 15 years. This should give lifelong protection, although boosters are given at or before special exposure, e.g. a wound (for tetanus) or travel abroad (for polio). Measles, mumps, and rubella (MMR) vaccine is given at 15 months of age, with a booster of rubella for girls aged 11 years. BCG vaccine should be given selectively to newborn babies whose families have a higher risk of tuberculosis—a close family history or immigration from Asia or Africa. Full details of these vaccinations are in the Department of Health's booklet 'Immunisation against infectious disease.

General Principles 5: The maintenance of herd immunity and measles vaccination

Measles vaccination has been given in Britain since 1968. The programme suffered in the early days through a lack of conviction that measles was serious enough to warrant prevention and because of problems in the supply of vaccine. The combination into a measles, mumps, and rubella vaccine has increased its popularity. There will be small outbreaks of measles, including some children who have been vaccinated, because the vaccine does not 'take' in about 4–5 per cent of recipients and because there is still a large pool of non-immune older children and young adults who dilute the herd immunity. Outbreaks should be investigated to check that the vaccine failure rate is no more than 5 per cent, and to find unvaccinated contacts who can be vaccinated as soon as possible.

Young adults

Vaccination after childhood is selective, for occupational, travel, or other risks. Often the risks of infection are remote and poorly documented, but the presence of any risk and the existence of a vaccine are deemed to be an indication. To the individual, the complications and costs of vaccination are small compared with a disease like hepatitis, meningococcal meningitis, or rabies. Doctors may gain financially, for example, in running travel clinics, so their advice is not unbiased.

The safest course is to follow the Department of Health booklet, as this tends to err on the side of caution. With specialist advice, there are some advances to be taken, as in using the intradermal route for some vaccines. A difficulty for the non-specialist is poor access to laboratory tests on antibody responses after modified courses of vaccination. The situation concerning unlicensed vaccines, e.g. Japanese B encephalitis and tick-borne encephalitis vaccines, which have had to be obtained on a named patient basis, is unsatisfactory. Neither the vaccinator nor the vaccinee have good information on what is being given, but both are responding to a vague recommendation that there is a risk which may be reduced by a vaccine. A general practitioner can make the preparation for overseas travel simpler for all parties by referring the person to a specialist travel clinic if there is one in the area. These clinics will often give a complete course of injections in one or two appointments.

A more worthwhile (in medical terms) activity is to protect young adults with vaccines against risks at home and at work. These are listed in Box 17.4.

Box 17.4: Vaccination guidelines for adults

BCG:

- People who are going to work in hospitals should have Heaf or Tine tests, and BCG if tuberculin negative.

Although BCG vaccine has been in the school health programme, some health authorities have stopped it and others may do so soon. A shortage of vaccine in 1989 and 1990 has left a cohort unvaccinated in most of Britain. Other European countries and the USA do not give BCG routinely.

Hepatitis B:

- For people whose sexual partners are, or are probably, infected;
- For health service staff in clinical practice;
- For patients and staff of residential institutions for the mentally handicapped.

Post vaccination antibodies should be checked, but 20 per cent of people will not sero-convert. All should be told of precautions against bloodborne infections.

Rubella:

- For women in antenatal and family planning clinics, if they are sero-negative.

A few will remain 'antibody-negative', but will in fact be immune. Those who have been vaccinated can be reassured.

Older people

Resistance to infection declines with age and infirmity, and this makes immunization a useful preventive tool for older people. Reminders about influenza vaccine are sent to general practitioners every autumn. In the past two years, influenza vaccine usage has been higher than the makers expected, which suggests that this vaccine was underused in the past. More than half of the cases of tetanus in recent years have been in older women who had never been vaccinated. It is more worthwhile to offer tetanus vaccine for women over the age of 50 years than to give men ten yearly boosters.

General Principles 6: Vaccination against pneumonia in older people and others at risk

Pneumococcal vaccine is being used in the USA for people over the age of 65 years, and for younger people with a higher than normal risk of pneumonia (sickle cell disease, asplenia, renal failure, and renal transplants, chronic chest disease, diabetes, liver disease, HIV infection). Pneumococcal vaccine is licensed in Britain, but has not been adopted for a national programme by the Department of Health. Nevertheless GPs should remember its availability for their patients in the high-risk groups listed.

Passive immunization

The words immunization and vaccination are often used interchangably, but the distinction is useful to remind us that temporary immunity can be conveyed by immunoglobin. The indications for this are relatively few, being inherited hypogammaglobilinaemias and specific exposures to certain infections. The duration of immunity is two to four months, depending on the dose. Immunoglobulin available in this country is a safe blood product, since its preparation has several steps which would prevent the transmission of blood-borne viruses.

Immunoglobulin is most commonly prescribed for travellers to countries with poor food and water hygiene. Its other uses are for people who are, or have been, already exposed to infection (see Box 17.5). The specific immunoglobulins are derived from blood donors with high antibody levels. They are scarce and are used only if the indications are definite.

Box 17.5: Guidelines on whom to vaccinate with immunoglobulin

1. Normal immunoglobulin for family contacts and outbreak control in hepatitis A.
2. Hepatitis-B-specific immunoglobulin for people exposed to the blood of a hepatitis B carrier.
3. Rabies-specific immunoglobulin for a person bitten by a rabid animal.
4. Tetanus-specific immunoglobulin for unimmunized patients with tetanus-prone wounds.
5. Varicella-Zoster-specific immunoglobulin for neonates whose mothers have chickenpox at the time of delivery, and for leukaemic and other immunosuppressed patients who become infected with chickenpox.
6. Normal immunoglobulin for leukaemic and other immunosuppressed children exposed to measles without prior vaccination.

Chemoprophylaxis

Chemoprophylaxis has limited usefulness, because of the development of antimicrobial resistance amongst microorganisms. The principles are to use antimicrobials for prophylaxis only when there is an indication proven by clinical trials, to keep the course of treatment as short as possible, and to restrict the use to as few people as possible.

Straightforward indications are long-term penicillin prophylaxis for children with rheumatic heart disease and perioperative prophylaxis for patients with abnormal heart values. There is a growing acceptance of perioperative prophylaxis in abdominal and pelvic surgery, and in prosthetic orthopaedic surgery. The hospital specialists usually arrange prophylaxis in these cases, but the GP should be aware in order to alert patients and consultants to drug allergies.

Chemoprophylaxis against malaria

Anti-malarials have the longest history, and drug resistance is a considerable problem. The choice is restricted to four agents, none of which is ideal. Chloroquine and proguanil are safe, but need to be taken in combination in most malarial areas and encounter varying degrees of resistance. Maloprim may cause bone-marrow damage, but is less likely to be nullified by resistant parasites. Mefloquin has more promise as an early treatment than as a prophylaxis, and is contra-indicated by epilepsy and psychiatric disorders. It is essential to warn travellers that anti-malarials are not completely effective, and to advise on how not to get bitten by mosquitoes.

Chemoprophylaxis against meningococcal meningitis

Although meningococcal meningitis is indication for chemoprophylaxis, the intention is to prevent spread by nasal carriers who may be in the family contacts of cases. The agent, rifampicin, taken twice a day for two days, does not treat early disease, so contacts should also be warned about the early signs of meningitis. Rifampicin prophylaxis is not well proven, but it is often more efficient for the hospital team to give rifampicin to the family on the ward than to refer them to their GP. GPs may be consulted by the patient's friends who ask for prophylaxis—careful explanations are more useful than prescriptions.

Hygiene and education

Hygiene and education look prosaic beside the conventional medical actions of prescribing drugs. Nevertheless they are essential in the control of infection. The incidences of tuberculosis and diphtheria were declining well before vaccines and antibiotics were introduced. Better housing, better diets, better standards of cleanliness—all elements of higher standards of living—are thought to have been important. There is greater certainty about the specific role of hygiene in the disposal of sewage in the elimination of cholera from Britain. Hygiene and education require further development to match the present-day problems.

General Principles 7: Simple hygiene measures in viral gastroenteritis

Viral gastroenteritis is endemic and common. There are a range of causative viruses, of which rotaviruses are the best understood. Rotavirus spread between young children in families and nurseries, fortunately conferring immunity on most. Small round structured viruses (SRSV) can be transmitted on uncooked foods (salads, fruit, and cold means) by people who are mildly ill. Hand-washing after using the lavatory and before preparing foods should be everyday practice, but needs to be emphasized for families with illness.

18 HIV and sexually transmitted diseases

Gorm Kirsch and Peter Anderson

Incidence of sexually transmitted diseases

Sexually transmitted diseases (STDs) are now outnumbered only by respiratory tract infections as a cause of reported communicable disease in England and Wales, and in Europe as a whole (Faculty of Public Health Medicine 1991). The apparent increase in the frequency of STDs that has been seen over the last decade is due not only to changes in incidence, but also to improvements in the range and availability of diagnostic tests fo these diseases, as well as to increases in public and professional awareness of STDs and their sequelae.

Much of the increase in awareness of STDs is a direct consequence of the advent of HIV infection and AIDS, which is now a major cause of mortality in the UK population. HIV infection will, in the absence of treatment, lead to the development of AIDS within ten years in at least 50 per cent of persons infected.

The sequelae of STDs include pelvic inflammatory disease (PID), ectopic pregnancy, infertility, congenital infections, developmental abnormalities, and carcinoma of the cervix, penis, and anus. Much of the burden of morbidity is experienced by women and young children. It is also apparent that STDs, such as genital herpes simplex infection, facilitate the transmission of HIV.

Adolescents appear to be at risk of acquiring STD. The proportion of attenders aged less than 20 years at genito-urinary medicine (GUM) clinics in England and Wales with syphilis and gonorrhoea increased slightly from 20 per cent in 1978 to 22 per cent in 1988. Increased susceptibility of adolescents to infection following exposure to *Chlamydia trachomatis*, and an increased risk among adolescents of developing cervical dysplasia and carcinoma following human papilloma virus (HPV) infection, has also been reported.

There were approximately 500 000 attendances at GUM clinics in England and Wales in 1988. The epidemiology of sexually transmitted diseases in England and Wales over the decade up to 1988 was dominated by a steady increase in the number of cases of STDs until 1986, particularly in women. In 1987, the total number of cases of STD seen in GUM clinics fell for the first time in over ten years; this fall was observed among men and women, and for most diseases, with the exception of genital warts. Within the trend for STDs as a whole, there were considerable variations by disease and by age and sex, with the highest rates of gonorrhoea being seen among the 16–24 year age-group for both men and women.

There was a steady fall in the number of new cases of syphilis and gonorrhoea seen in GUM clinics between 1978 and 1988, and an overall rise in the number of cases of non-specific genital infection, genital herpes, and genital warts. Greater increases in case numbers have been seen for women than for men, and greater reductions in the rate of gonorrhoea and syphilis were seen among attenders aged 25 years and over than among those aged less than 25 years.

HIV/AIDS is arguably the greatest new threat to public health this century. It has been estimated that about 5000 new cases of AIDS will be reported in homosexual men in England during 1989–93. Predictions of numbers of cases acquired by transmission through heterosexual intercourse and injecting drug use are more difficult, but it is possible that by 1993 over half the new cases could be in these two categories compared with only 7 per cent of reports in the first nine months of 1989.

By the end of December 1990 there had been a total of 3817 reported cases of AIDS in England, of whom 55 per cent had died. There were 12985 known HIV antibody positive people, of whom 1099 were female. The figures for those known to be HIV positive are likely to be substantially less than the true number.

AIDS cases in homosexual and bisexual men still account for 81 per cent of the total. However, the rate of increase in new cases amongst this group during 1990 was only 46 per cent compared with an 82 per cent increase in cases acquired by heterosexual intercourse during the same year and an even greater increase in the number of people infected by contaminated drug-injecting equipment. Cases amongst women increased by 119 per cent, rising from 37 per cent at the end of December 1989 to 81 per cent by December 1990.

As with AIDS cases, there is evidence of rapid growth in the number of people infected with HIV through heterosexual intercourse. Reports in this group increased by 65 per cent during 1990, compared with 20 per cent for homosexual or bisexual men. Just under half the infected heterosexual people are women.

Preventing sexually transmitted diseases

Risk reduction

The most efficacious means of reducing the risk of acquiring HIV or other sexually transmitted diseases through sexual contact is either abstinence from sexual relations or maintenance of a mutually monogamous sexual relationship with an uninfected partner (Faculty of Public Health Medicine of the Royal College of Physicians 1991). If the infection status of the partner is uncertain, sexual relations should be avoided, particularly with persons at increased risk for HIV infection (e.g. homosexual and bisexual men, intravenous drug users). The prevalence of HIV infection in heterosexual partners of persons in high-risk categories may be as high as 11 per cent, and as many as 60 per cent of heterosexual partners of HIV-infected individuals may be seropositive. Risk is directly related to the number of sexual partners, in part because of the difficulty of obtaining adequate information on risk status from each partner.

Certain sexual practices may also influence the risk of infection. Among homosexual men, for example, receptive anal intercourse has been repeatedly implicated as a principal risk factor for HIV infection, and other practices that increase rectal trauma may have a similar role. Conversely, some sexual practices, such as using latex condoms and spermicides, may reduce the risk of infection. Condoms have been shown in the laboratory to prevent transmission of *Chlamydia trachomatis*, herpes simplex virus, trichmonas, cytomegalovirus, and HIV. Although further data are needed on the efficacy of latex condoms in actual practice, there is epidemiological evidence that persons who use condoms correctly are at decreased risk of acquiring gonococcal and nongonococcal urethritis and HIV infection. Even under optimal conditions, however, condoms are not always efficacious in preventing transmission. Condom failures occur at an estimated rate of 10–15 per cent, either as a result of product failure (e.g. breakage) or as a result of incorrect or inconsistent use. Natural membrane condoms are more permeable than latex condoms to passage of HIV and other sexually transmitted organisms such as herpes virus and they are less uniform than latex condoms. Errors on the part of users, however, are thought to be the most likely cause of condom failure. Incorrect use has been shown to limit the effectiveness of condoms in preventing gonorrhoea and presumably also permits passage of more dangerous organisms such as HIV.

The use of spermicides, along with condoms, has been proposed as a means of further reducing the risk of infection. One of the spermicidal agents that has been investigated, nonoxynol-9, has been shown to have *in vitro* activity against herpes simplex virus, hepatitis B, and HIV. It also has clinical efficacy in reducing risk of gonorrhoea and chlamydial infection in women. In many clinical studies, however, spermicides were used in combination with condoms or diaphragms, and therefore it is unclear which intervention or combination of interventions was directly responsible for the outcome. There is also inadequate information on the effectiveness of spermicides inserted in condoms if the condoms rupture; sub-inhibitory concentrations of spermicide would presumably be more likely if condom rupture occurs in the rectum (or in the vagina in the absence of supplemental vaginal application of spermicide).

Additional measures to reduce the risk of infection with HIV and hepatitis B include avoiding the use of intravenous drugs or unsterilized needles and syringes. The characteristics of drug use often make prompt discontinuation of intravenous drug use difficult. Drug management programmes, such as methadone maintenance clinics, can be effective in some patients, but many drug users lack access to such facilities or return to their habit following treatment. Even in persons who continue to use intravenous drugs, morbidity and mortality from HIV, hepatitis B, and bacterial endocarditis could be reduced by using sterilized needles and syringes. AIDS is the leading cause of death in this population, and even a modest reduction in risk could have significant public health implications. Methods for obtaining uncontaminated drug equipment include purchasing sterilized equipment, obtaining free products through distribution programmes, and cleaning used equipment with a bleach solution.

Counselling

There have been few studies examining the effectiveness of physicians in influencing the sexual behaviour of patients. Studies of clinic-based educational programmes, which in some cases have included physician counselling as a component, have culminated in reporting of an increased rate of return for test-of-cure and reduced incidence of certain sexually transmitted diseases, but these studies involved select populations and provided little evidence of change in sexual behaviour (US Preventive Services Task Force 1989). Other successful measures have included distribution of free condoms to male adolescents and of bleach products to clean drug-injection equipment, but these items were not distributed by physicians. Sexual behaviour appears to have changed significantly in recent years as a result of increased public awareness of AIDS. Homosexual and bisexual men report fewer high-risk sexual practices. Behaviour may also be changing in heterosexual populations living in high-risk areas and in some intravenous drug users.

There is also evidence from recent surveys that behaviour is not changing dramatically in certain population groups, such as adolescents and college students, despite increased knowledge of the health risks associated with high-risk sexual practices. A number of factors may account for this reluctance to change behaviour. Compliance with the proper use of condoms and spermicides can be affected by perceptions of inconvenience, concerns about sexual spontaneity, and cultural attitudes. Prostitutes and drug addicts, who have special dependency on high-risk behaviours, face added difficulties in changing behaviour.

Clinicians may provide ineffective counselling or no counselling if they have inadequate historical data on the patient's sexual and drug use behaviour. A complete sexual history is therefore important as a prelude to any form of effective counselling to prevent sexually transmitted diseases. Many clinicians do not, however, take an adequate sexual history.

Clinical intervention

Clinicians should take a complete sexual and drug use history on adult patients. Sexually active patients should receive complete information on their risk for acquiring sexually transmitted diseases. They should be advised that abstaining from sex or maintaining a mutually faithfully monogamous sexual relationship with a partner known to be uninfected are the most effective strategies to prevent infection with HIV or other sexually transmitted diseases. Patients should be advised against sexual activity with individuals whose infection status is uncertain. A non-reactive HIV test does not rule out infection if the sexual partner has not been monogamous and if monogamous, with an infected person for at least six months before the test. Patients who choose to engage in sexual activities with multiple partners or with persons who may be infected should be advised to use a condom at each encouter and to avoid anal intercourse. Women should be informed of the potential risks of HIV infection during pregnancy. Persons who use intravenous drugs should be encouraged to enrol in a drug treatment programme, warned against sharing drug equipment and using unsterilized syringes and needles, and given sources for uncontaminated injection equipment or refered to community programmes with this information. Patients should be offered testing in accordance with local recommendations on screening for infection with HIV.

Condoms need not be recommended to prevent infection in longstanding mutually monogamous relationships in which neither partner uses intravenous drugs or is infected with HIV. Those patients who need to use condoms should be informed that they do not provide complete protection against infection and to be effective must be used in accordance with the guidelines shown in Box 18.1

Box 18.1: Guidelines for safe use of condoms

- Latex condoms, rather than natural membrane condoms, should be used. Torn condoms, those in damaged packages, or those with signs of age (brittle, sticky, discoloured) should not be used.
- The condom should be put on an erect penis, before any intimate contact, and should be unrolled completely to the base.
- A space should be left at the tip of the condom to collect semen; air pockets in the space should be removed by pressing the air out towards the base.
- Water-based lubricants should be used. Those made with petroleum jelly, mineral oil, cold cream, and other oil-based lubricants should not be applied because they may damage the condom.

- Insertion of nonoxynol-9 in the condom increases protection, but vaginal or anal application in addition to condom use is likely to provide greater protection.
- If a condom breaks, it should be replaced immediately.
- After ejaculation, and while the penis is still erect, the penis should be withdrawn while carefully holding the condom against the base of the penis so that the condom remains in place.
- Condoms should not be reused.

Concerns for general practice

Maintaining confidentiality

Good preventive efforts on HIV infection must begin with the basics. The full confidence of both patients and staff requires of the practice the very highest standards. Because of the social stigma often attached to people with HIV infection, or population groups perceived to be at particular risk, it is essential that GPs and their teams do their utmost to ensure that all information that comes into, circulates within, and leaves the practice be handled in such a way that patients will always feel that it is being used in their best interest. Among the areas that individual practice teams need to consider are the following:

1. Information entering the practice:
   - Who sees it? The receptionist, nurse, or doctor?
   - Where does it wait until being passed on, i.e. can 'unauthorised' individuals, for example other patients or staff, read it?
   - Where and how is information recorded, and by whom?
2. Information within, and being used by, the practice:
   - Where and how is it held—paper, notes, computer, combination, patient-held?
   - How is it retrieved? by user, secretary/receptionist, nurse?
   - How is it returned? Where does it await refiling?
3. Information held, but not in current use:
   - Where and how held? Separate archives or main notes?
   - Who has access? Anyone with access to main notes?
4. Information leaving the practice:
   - Where does it go?
   - Who is getting it—system for checking enquiries, for example, checking enquiries from hospital by phoning back?
   - How will it be used?
   - Who authorises release?

Clearly, although recognizing the importance of good confidentiality for all patients, the amount of information moving through a typical GP surgery makes the task quite a challenging one. In conjunction with a review of the way in which information is handled, all staff need to be reminded of what confidentiality means and why it is important. Receptionists, if consulted, often have many valuable suggestions about how work practices could be subtly changed to ensure a better system. Team-work, and making full-practice decisions, is vital when it comes to confidentiality. In many cases, discussing with the patient what will happen to their notes can prevent problems.

Controlling infection

Ensuring that staff feel confident about their health and safety is another fundamental issue which any practice considering its approach to HIV prevention must take into account. Given the different levels of education, information, and advice, it should never be assumed that all staff feel confident about the control of infection. Once again, policies and practice within the teams should be reviewed and all staff (including non-clinical staff such as receptionists, and cleaners) should be involved in discussions, and asked their opinion.

Emergencies

There are few real emergencies in HIV, and many apparent ones. Emergency services (police, ambulance, and fire) all have some training in how to cope with blood spillages (Box 18.2) from people who may be HIV or hepatitis B positive. Needle-stick injuries in which health staff may be exposed to HIV positive blood should be dealt with promptly (see Box 18.3).

Box 18.2: Guidelines for the management of blood spillages

- All spillages should be dealt with immediately and latex gloves should be worn.
- If appropriate to the contaminated surfaces, a solution of 10 per cent bleach in water should be used to wipe the area clean. On other surfaces (e.g. carpets) spillage should be allowed to dry (which will destroy HIV), and a cleaning powder can then be used.
- On washable items household detergent in a normal household washing machine will inactivate the virus.

Box 18.3: Guidelines for the management of needle-stick injuries

1. Find out what happened.
2. Clean the wound.
3. Discover, if possible, the name of the person believed to be HIV positive and try to check the information.
4. Ask the injured person if he or she is willing to be tested for HIV antibodies, and contact the virology laboratory for an urgent test. But seroconversion after HIV infection may take at least 3 months, so testing should preferably be delayed for this time.
5. If exposure to HIV seems to be a real possibility a short course (six weeks) of zidovudine may be helpful, although this is an unproven prophylaxis.

References and further reading

Faculty of Public Health Medicine of the Royal Colleges of Physicians (1991). *UK levels of health.* Faculty of Public Health Medicine, London.

Moss, A. (1992). *AIDS and HIV (Practical guides for general practice).* Oxford University Press.

US Preventive Services Task Forces (1989). *Guide to clinical preventive services.* Williams and Wilkins, Baltimore.

19 Preventing mental ill-health

Andrew Markus

Introduction

The definition of mental ill-health is not precise; hence the wide range of reported prevalence of mental illness. Whether a patient's feeling of being unwell is labelled illness depends on a variety of factors, including:

- the patient's own perception of good health;
- the health professional's definition of disease;
- the ability of the health professional to identify disease when it is present;
- society's definition of what is normal.

It also depends on the organization of health care; in countries without the 'gatekeeper' type of primary care which exists in the UK, everyone referring themselves to a psychiatist would, by definition, be labelled a 'psychiatric case'. In such countries, prevention in this context might include intervention by a primary care physician which prevents a patient being referred to a psychiatrist. The use of validated screening questionnaires such as the General Health Questionnaire (GHQ) suggests a prevalence of mental ill-health in the UK of around 25 per cent but the figure varies with age, sex, and social class. Moreover, it is important to remember that the GHQ does not identify people with psychotic illness or those with personality problems.

The achievement of mental health requires a satisfactory balance between genetic endowment and social interaction, the most important aspect of which is the ambience of family life. Although there is evidence, for example from studies of identical twins reared apart, that genetic factors play a part in the development of schizophrenia and other forms of mental illness, influencing mental ill-health by genetic manipulation is not yet possible.

Models for preventing mental ill-health

As in other aspects of prevention, conceptual models can be useful when considering the prevention of mental illness.

The *disease model* approach starts with the study of illness and attempts to identify the causal factors which it may be possible to influence. While it may be possible to identify a number of such factors, it is likely that these will interact in various ways, so it is difficult to disentangle and influence them independently. However, using such a multifactorial disease model for prevention, it may be possible to identify those patients particularly at risk. For example, if bereavement is found to predispose to depression, the risk group, i.e. those most recently bereaved, would be very large. If, however, lack of a supportive network was also found to be influential, the 'at-risk' group would be smaller and would be more easily targeted.

The *health model* approach, on the other hand, assumes that if a number of people are exposed to the same risk factors some will become ill while others will remain healthy. This suggests that there are protective factors at work and, by looking at populations with respect to individuals' everyday lives, it may then be possible to identify these protective factors. By concentrating on the enhancement of these protective factors, facilitation of good health may be achieved and disease avoided. Such protective factors include the enhancement of supportive communities, reduction in social inequality, and improved access to health care.

Ideally, these two models need to be combined, not only to reduce the incidence of disease but to increase individuals' ability to withstand it. But it must also be emphasized that the part health professionals can play in the prevention of mental ill-health is necessarily limited.

Approaches to prevention

As in all forms of prevention of disease, three types can be identified: primary, secondary, and tertiary prevention.

Primary prevention aims to reduce the incidence of the disorder by identifying its causes and avoiding or removing these. In the mental health field, measures that seek to ameliorate the affects of mother–child separation in childhood are a good example, as it is known that such separation may contribute to emotional problems later on. Any involvement by the primary care team in improvement of social support within the local community will also assist the primary prevention of mental ill-health.

Secondary prevention involves the identification of incipient or hidden disease followed by appropriate action to prevent it developing to a harmful stage. In the mental health field, secondary prevention includes any activity which allows individuals to get help for problems which, if allowed to persist could develop into mental illness. General practitioners are often in a position to recognize distress and by appropriate help to prevent the development of full-blown illness.

Tertiary prevention involves measures aimed at avoiding deterioration or recurrence in people who already have illness. In the mental health field, the follow-up of patients who have already had a schizophrenic episode provides an example of tertiary prevention. This may include continuation of drug treatment as part of continuing and team care.

Team care

Because of their location in the community and their long-term relationships with patients, general practitioners are often in a position to help individuals in relation to mental illness as well as to influence the local, and sometimes the national, environment.

Patients coming the see the doctor usually present with a problem or problems. It is one of the general practitioner's tasks to elucidate clauses and, very often, in spite of a physical presentation (such as backache) the problem may largely be psychological in origin. In every consultation, there is a need to make an appraisal in psychological and social, as well as physical, terms. Doctors differ in their ability to make such appraisals, and it has been shown by Goldberg (1982) that this skill can be improved by training. Medical behaviours which improve the accuracy of psychological assessment and which can be significantly improved by training are listed in Box 19.1.

Box 19.1 Medical behaviours which relate to accuracy of psychological assessment and which can be improved by training (after Goldberg 1982)

Start of inteview:
- making eye contact with patient;
- clarification of presenting complaint (through open questions).

Form of 'problem-solving' questions:
- proportion directive (rather than closed);
- use of directive questions when dealing with physical symptoms;
- focusing on the present rather than the past.

Some special techniques:
- sensitivity to verbal cues relating to psychological distress;
- sensitivity to non-verbal cues;
- ability to deal with over-talkative patients.

But, as with other aspects of primary care, a team approach is important in the prevention of mental ill-health—not only in identifying the development of problems, but in minimizing their harmful effects. The primary health care team has much relevant expertise available in health visitors, practice nurses, community nurses, social workers, counsellors, clinical psychologists, community psychiatric nurses, and others. But in the mental health field in particular, personalities may matter more than professional labels, and roles may overlap. For example, a male social worker may be more helpful than a female counsellor for one patient, and for another a female health visitor more helpful than a male community psychiatric nurse. It is a matter of 'horses for courses', and demarcation disputes within teams should be avoided.

Life events

There is much evidence that particular life events may produce psychological reactions resulting in consultations with general practitioners. Whatever the form of the presentation, the common feature is that the patient is going through a psycho-social transition which involves relinquishing one set of assumptions about the world and the adoption of another. Individuals may be particularly vulnerable at such times but, through the process of readjusting their view of the world, may learn coping skills which make them better able to withstand future stresses. The general practitioner is frequently in a position to help at these times and may thereby contribute to the prevention of mental illness. Examples of psycho-social transitions are illustrated in Box 19.2.

Box 19.2: Examples of psycho-social transitions

Childhood
- Loss of or separation from parents.
- Loss of close relatives or friends.
- Loss of familiar environment, e.g. hospital admission.

Adolescence
- Separation from parents or home.
- Personal problems, e.g. relationship break-up.
- Sexual identification.

Young adults
- Marriage
- Pregnancy (especially the first).
- Birth of a handicapped child.
- Marital breakdown.
- Loss of job.

Older adults
- Retirement.
- Loss of mobility.
- Bereavement.
- Loss of familiar environment, e.g. entering old people's home.

For many, life is full of stressful events and it may be the acuteness of onset or the cumulative effect which provokes breakdown. For example, a mother may cope with several children in a damp house and only break down when she hears about the illness of her father.

Of course, many people cope with life events without outside help and whether mental ill-health is precipitated depends not only on the nature of the life event but on the vulnerability of the individual. If the life event is major, if it is of a type which has previously lead to unresolved problems, or if there is no time for preparation, it is more likely to lead to the breakdown of coping mechanisms. Vulnerability is enhanced by belonging to a low socio-economic group, having several small young children at home, being unemployed, living in overcrowded conditions, and having low self-esteem.

By taking these factors into account, general practitioners can identify more precisely those patients on whom efforts to help should be concentrated. If the life event is predictable, intervention may be possible before the life event, in the form of 'anticipatory guidance'–or by crisis management during or after the event. The types of intervention available are outlined in Table 19.1.

Table 19.1 Types of intervention

Education	Competence Problem-solving skills Self efficacy
Anticipatory guidance	Accurate information to patient Time to digest information Encouragement of patient to react emotionally Provision of reassurance
Crisis intervention	Minimize impact Relief from everyday duties Encouragement of emotional expression Encouragement to seek new directions
Therapy	Early diagnosis and treatment of pathological reaction Referral to health visitor, counsellor, social worker, psychiatrist, etc.

Childhood and adolescence

Time brings many surprises in general practice, perhaps none more pleasing than the emergence of a happy, well-balanced young person from a fraught family background. But life is not often so kind, and general practitioners are well placed, together with the various members of their primary care teams, to ameliorate the harmful influences abounding in some families.

There are two main patterns of psychological malfunction which occur in childhood. One is characterized by anxiety, either general or specific, to certain situations. This may result in preoccupation with physical symptoms such as abdominal pain, with school refusal, or with generalized social withdrawal. The other pattern is associated with antisocial behaviour, such as stealing, aggressive behaviour, and truanting. Although there is some overlap between these patterns, they appear to be generated by different family dynamics, and their origins will be considered separately here.

Anxiety states are most commonly caused by an insecure mother–child relationship. This is most likely to occur if:

- the mother is alone and has no close, supportive relationship;
- the pregnancy has been complicated;
- there has been a previous obstetric disaster which makes the child especially precious;
- there is guilt surrounding the circumstances of conception.

Situations such as these tend to make the mother overprotective and thus interfere with normal development of independence in the child. Any new challenge, especially if it involves separation from the mother, may cause anxiety, transferred from mother to child. This results in clinging behaviour so often seen in the surgery when a child refuses to be examined, and this should act as a warning to the general practitioner that all is not well. Later, battles may develop over going to school, and the lack of confidence and independence may lead to interpersonal problems in adolescence. Such children are probably also more likely to develop anxiety states and phobic reactions when they grow up—and so the cycle repeats itself.

Delinquency and *antisocial behaviour* arise from a low tolerance of frustration. This leads the young person to resort to aggressive behaviour to get what he or she wants, and a tendency not to trust other people means that making close relationships becomes difficult. Lack of warmth and consistency in parent–child relationship is probably the most important factor contributing to this. The child may be 'difficult' after birth, crying a lot, and sleeping irregularly. The parents may have problems of their own which reduce their ability to tolerate such behaviour, and the scene is set for parental rejection, child abuse, or just withdrawal of nurture which leaves these children lonely and frustrated. Some end up in childrens' homes and may then have a succession of carers with whom they are unable to develop an individual and close relationship.

Prevention of these disorders has important implications for general practice. In consultations with patients with young families, general practitioners should be aware of clues suggesting possible problems in the future and should be prepared to provide appropriate help, whether a listening ear, information, or advice. Sometimes there is a need to be proactive, trying to reduce the impact of anticipated events and at other times to be reactive, responding to current difficulties.

For example, the young girl who may be at risk of getting pregnant may need to be helped with contraceptive advice. Couples who are thinking of starting a family need to be offered advice which should cover not only the physical changes to be expected during pregnancy and relevant aspects of lifestlye, such as the avoidance of smoking, but also the alteration in the dynamics of their relationship which is bound to occur when a baby arrives, especially the first.

Again, at the post-natal visit, problems should be anticipated and parents helped to cope in a way which will enhance their ability to manage. The 'difficult' baby needs to be identified and the parents reassured that all babies have personalities of their own and this doesn't mean that the child is naughty and needs to be punished. It is often helpful at this stage to see the parents together, to explore their health beliefs and their views on being parents, and to encourage them to work together. It is easy for problems over beliefs as to how children should be brought up to divide a couple, especially if there is a dominating grandparent in the background. The fluctuating mood of the post-natal mother also needs anticipating and accepting by all parties, and the frank post-natal depression identified and treated early. Attention needs to be paid to the bonding which develops between mother and child, and separation kept to a minimum. The classic work of Bowlby (1988) has shown that children who are separated from their mothers during early childhood, for instance through hospital admission, are more likely to exhibit symptoms of anxiety later in life. General practitioners need to try to reduce such separation to a minimum and to explain to all involved the reasons why they should do this; the health visitor can be an invaluable ally in these matters.

It is necessary to be aware of the development of over-close mother-child relationships which are likely to impede the emergence of independence in the child. Always treating the child as an individual in the consulting room is helpful; so many consultations about children take place over their heads. Children, too, bring an agenda to the consultation, and have anxieties about their illness which they want answered. In this way, young people may come to trust their general practitioner and build up relationships which can help to avoid trouble in adolescence or later life.

One way of building up this trust and marking the event of entering into adult life is to set aside time for a more formal consultation with young people who are around the age of 16 (such consultations are sometimes labelled as 'adolescent MOTs'). This can be done on an opportunistic basis within an ordinary consultation, or by calling in the 16-year-olds from the practice register–or by a combination of both.

A number of issues can be covered in such a consultation, of which perhaps the most important is to emphasize that both legally and ethically they are now adults and therefore can be offered a higher degree of confidentiality than when they were younger. There is, of course, no such thing as absolute confidentiality in ordinary medical practice, and the interests of society may outweigh those of the individual. But 16-year-olds can certainly be offered the same degree of confidentiality as their parents can expect. It can be made clear to them that, just as their parents' problems would never be discussed with them, so things they have discussed would never be told to their parents.

Patterns of behaviour are laid down in childhood and adolescence. Some families can only express distress in physical terms. These are the families whose children are brought to the doctor with a story of recurrent stomach-ache, headache, or tiredness. If these complaints are given a label by the doctor which implies a physical disorder, when the real problem may be, for instance, upset at the parents' marital squabbling, the young person's tendency to try to express all pain in physical terms is reinforced. By accepting emotional problems as 'real', the doctor can encourage young people not to mask their feelings.

There is some evidence that if children with dyslexia (specific reading retardation) can be identified early, remedial action can prevent the emergence of associated and emotional problems later. Such children are often highly intelligent and become very frustrated when they fall behind their peers at school. The doctor may be in a position to arrange for psychological assessment and special tuition at an early age, and so help avoid later problems.

Adult life

Anxiety and depression account for the majority of adult general practice consultations in the mental health field and early and appropriate management of these may prevent later problems.

Anxiety and depression are emotions felt by most normal people. There are times, however, when both these emotions become difficult to cope with and these are the very times when patients may consult their doctors. Frequently the two are present at the same time. Anxiety states may be generalized or may relate to specific situations or objects when they are labelled as 'phobias'. Depressive states may be relatively mild, differing from sadness only in minor degree, or may be much more severe, involving various physical manifestations such as loss of energy, appetite, and libido, as well as disturbed sleep with early waking and diurnal variation of mood.

The scope for prevention by the general practitioner and the primary care team is limited but counselling, particularly in relation to life events, and advice on stress management, may be helpful. The social aspect of problems should always be elucidated and social interventions may be more important than strictly medical ones.

Suicide

About two-thirds of patients attempting suicide consult a general practitioner in the month before the attempt and a similar proportion give warning to someone of their intent (Hawton and Catalan 1982). Moreover, a substantial proportion of such patients have been prescribed psychotropic drugs by their general practitioner before the attempt. There must therefore be scope for prevention in primary care if such 'at-risk' patients can be identified.

In addition to genuine suicide attempts which are often related to depressive states and are commonest in older males, the condition of 'parasuicide' is also recognized; this is deliberate self-harm, without suicidal intent, and occurs usually on impulse, commonly in young females.

Parasuicide has been shown to be related to:

- disturbed relationship with a key individual, frequently following a quarrel;
- poor social condition;
- high unemployment;
- large family size;
- early parental death;
- past criminal or anti-social record.

Associated factors include alcoholism, epilepsy, and drug addiction.

General practitioners should make assessment of suicidal risk part of every consultation with a patient in a high-risk group or situation. It is always better to ask someone whether they have contemplated suicide rather than fear 'putting thoughts into a patient's head'. Psychotropic drug prescribing to high-risk patients should be avoided or, if necessary, a responsible person should be asked to look after the medication. Potentially suicidal patients should be given open access to a doctor or other counselling agency. If the doctor can build up a relationship of trust, it is more likely that at times of crisis help may be sought and accepted and the opportunity to prevent self-destructive behaviour thereby enhanced.

Old age

The predominant mental illness in the elderly is senile dementia. This is an irreversible condition of reduced cerebral function resulting from organic damage to the brain. It causes loss of memory for recent events, slowing and poverty of thought processes, impaired judgement, and a tendency to disorientation. Whilst there is no evidence that the progress of the pathological processes can be influenced, the effects can be aggravated by a number of circumstances which may be alterable and allow some scope for prevention. Anaemia, hypothermia, malnutrition, accidental injury, and various drugs in high dosage may all be contributory factors which are amenable to change.

However, the commonest and most distressing cause is probably environmental change; moving confused people away from a familiar environment such as their home, into hospital, an old person's home, or even on holiday may upset their tenuous hold on reality. Environmental change needs to be reduced to a minimum. Confused elderly patients are better treated in one place, and if they are ill at home it may be better to arrange for help from a district nurse, home help, and other agencies rather than admit them to hospital. Family members and other carers are more likely to cooperate with such plans if their needs are also recognized and attended to. It may be possible to keep an elderly person at home by arranging regular visits by members of the primary care team, or by volunteers, or by arranging for day hospital or 'floating bed' care on a regular basis. This may make all the difference to whether or not carers are prepared to go on looking after a trying patient in the community. If an elderly person is noted to be deteriorating, and is likely to require a permanent move away from familiar surroundings at some time, it is best to arrange this early while the patient is still able to understand what is going on and able to adapt to the new environment.

Prevention: its implications in practice

Traditionally, the doctor's role has been to respond to the patient's presenting complaint. Some would still argue that to go beyond this is to infringe patient autonomy. The present day philosophy of general practice, however, emphasizes its role in whole person care on a continuing basis for individuals and a defined community. This care includes anticipatory, i.e. preventive, care as well as the management of new problems and the continuing care of existing ones.

There is evidence that such comprehensive care is what patients increasingly expect from their doctors and that the inclusion of preventive care, whether physical or psycho-social, into general practice consultations is thought to be appropriate by patients. How to do this is a skill general practitioners need to develop if consultations are to retain a patient-centred approach and not be dominated by the doctor's agenda.

It might be argued that to try to cover the prevention of mental ill-health in the course of ordinary consultations is unrealistic, bearing in mind the time constraints of general practice. However, if such ill-health is really prevented, or just made less serious, it is likely that, overall, time will be saved. It should also be remembered that general practitioners are likely to know so much about their patients already that a simple question, such as 'How are things in general?', will give an idea of whether any serious trouble is brewing.

If intervention seems appropriate, simple counselling in which the doctor helps the patient to look at emerging problems, discusses possible strategies, helps to reframe thoughts, and tries to help patients increase their own coping skills may be all that is necessary. On some occasions when problems are identified, the doctor will need to make arrangements either to see the patient on another occasion when more time is available, or to involve other health care professionals. Thus referral may be made for individual treatment to a health visitor or counsellor, to a group run by a member of the primary care team or by someone outside, to some other agency, or to a psychiatrist.

Conclusion

The approach advocated in this chapter requires the development of a wider 'primary care team' in each practice with consequent challenges for organization and communication. Areas of confidentiality will need to be defined, access to records agreed, referral procedures drawn up, and so on. Members of the team will need frequent opportunities to meet each other, both informally and formally, and to share the burden of such taxing work. The challenge is a major one, but the potential rewards in professional satisfaction and patient well-being are considerable.

References and further reading

Bowlby, J. (1988). *A secure base. Clinical applications of attachment theory.* Routledge, London. (A series of essays which gives a good introduction to Bowlby's thinking.)

Brown, G. W. and Harris, T. (1978). *Social origins of depression.* Tavistock, London.

Caplan, G. (1964). *Principles of preventive psychiatry.* Basic Books, New York.

Erikson, E. H. (1968). *Identity, youth and crisis.* Faber and Faber, London.

Goldberg, D. (1982). In *Psychiatry in general practice*, (ed. A. Clare and M. Lader), pp. 35–41. Academic, London.

Goldberg, D. and Huxley, P. (1980). *Mental illness in the community.* Tavistock, London.

Hawton, K. and Catalan, J. (1982). *Attempted suicide.* Oxford University Press.

Newton, J. (1988). *Preventing mental illness.* Routledge and Kegan Paul, London. (The best introduction to the subject including a summary of research work in this field.)

Royal College of General Practitioners (1981). Prevention of psychiatric disorders in general practice, *Report from General Practice* No. 20. Royal College of General Practitioners, London.

Some organizations offering advice and information about emotional and mental illness health problems

- For young people:
  Brook Advisory Centres
  153A East Street
  London SE17 2SD
- Marital counselling:
  Relate
  Herbert Gray College
  Little Church Street
  Rugby CV21 3AP

  Catholic Marriage Advisory Council
  15 Lansdowne Road
  Holland Park
  London W11 3AJ
- Bereavement counselling:
  CRUSE
  Cruse House
  126 Sheen Road
  Richmond
  Surrey TW9 1UR
- General:
  Mental Health Foundation
  8 Hallam Street
  London W1N 6HD

  MIND (National Association for Mental Health)
  22 Harley Street
  London W1N 2ED

  The Samaritans
  17 Uxbridge Road
  Slough
  Bucks SL1 1SN

Appendix: The New UK general practice contract

Godfrey Fowler

Primary health care

Primary health care services are the frontline of the National Health Service. They include all those services provided outside hospital by family doctors, dentists, retail pharmacists, and opticians—the 'family practitioner services'—and by community nurses, midwives, health visitors, and other professions allied to medicine–'community health services'. These services deal with over 90 per cent of the contacts that people have with the health service.

On an average day, about three-quarters of a million people are seen by their family doctor and about 5 million visit a local pharmacy. About another 100 000 are visited by nurses or other health professionals, working in the community.

These primary health care services account for about 30 per cent of total expenditure on the National Health Service.

The Government's review

With the publication in April 1986 of *Primary health care: an agenda for discussion*, the Government launched what was claimed as the first comprehensive review of primary health care services in the 40 years since the NHS Act was passed in 1946.

Although acknowledging the development of services in general practice for the prevention of ill-health and the promotion of good health, emphasis in this review was placed on the increasing scope for doing more, for example, early detection of hypertension, in the prevention of coronary heart disease, by advice on smoking, diet and physical fitness. It also acknowledged that:

> Prevention is not solely for doctors. Nurses generally, as well as health visitors, and other members of primary care teams have important roles to play.

In November 1987, the Government's 'programme' for improving primary health care *Promoting better health* was published. In this programme, further emphasis was put on the role of primary health care in preventing disease and it was stated that 'there remains a massive amount which could be done to reduce the incidence of disease' (see Box A.1). In the programme, it was stated that, 'The Government intends positively to encourage family doctors and primary health care teams to increase their contribution to the promotion of good health'. The Report of the Social Services Committee included comment on the Government's plans:

> few, if any, commentators would disagree with the premise that the next challenge for the NHS, and one especially for primary health care, is to shift the emphasis from an illness service to a health service, offering to help to prevent disease and disability.

The new general practice contract

The general practice contact and revised terms of service, introduced in April 1990, make it clear that health promotion and illness prevention now

Box A.1: The potential for prevention

Cancer:
- most women who die from cancer of the cervix have never had a cervical smear.

Obesity:
- a quarter of young people are overweight.

Measles:
- there were 90 000 cases in 1986 and over 1000 hospital admissions.

Alcohol misuse:
- alcohol is a factor in 1 in 3 attendances by men at hospital accident and emergency departments.

Drug misuse:
- the number of addicts newly notified in 1986 exceeded 5000.

Smoking:
- 100 000 deaths each year are caused by smoking;
- about 500 million working days are lost;
- about 400 million pounds in NHS treatment costs are attributable to smoking.

Dental disease:
- children under 16 have some two and a quarter million teeth extracted and six and half million fillings each year.

Coronary heart disease:
- 180 000 deaths occur each year and an estimated 38 million working days are lost in Britain.

fall within the definition of general medical services. Previously, a general practitioner had been required to 'render to his patients all necessary and appropriate personal and medical services of the type usually provided by general practitioners'. The new requirements include the following.

1. Giving advice, where appropriate, to a patient in connection with the patient's general health, and in particular about the significance of diet, exercise, the use of tobacco, the consumption of alcohol, and the misuse of drugs and solvents.
2. Offering to patients consultations and, where appropriate, physical examination for the purpose of identifying, or reducing the risk of, disease or injury.
3. Offering to patients, where appropriate, vaccination or immunization against measles, mumps, rubella, pertussis, poliomyelitis, diphtheria, and tetanus.

Newly registered patients

As part of the extended obligation to provide services concerned with the prevention of ill-health and the promotion of good health, the general practitioner is now required to offer all newly registered patients, aged 5 years or over, a 'health check', to be carried out by the doctor or other appropriate member of the primary health care team. The requirements are to:

1. Seek details from the patient about his or her medical history and, as far as it may be relevant to the patient's medical history, about those of consanguineous family, in respect of:
   - illness, immunization, allergies, hereditary conditions, medication, and tests carried out for breast or cervical cancer;
   - social factors (including employment, housing, and family circumstances) that may affect his or her health;
   - factors of lifestyle (including diet, exercise, use of tobacco, consumption of alcohol, and misuse of drugs or solvents) that may affect his or her health; and
   - current state of health.
2. Offer to undertake a physical examination of the patient, comprising:
   - measurement of height, weight, and blood pressure; and
   - the taking of a urine sample for subsequent analysis to identify the presence of albumin and glucose.
3. Record in the patient's medical records, findings arising out of the details supplied by, and any examination of, the patient.
4. Assess whether and, if so, in what manner and to what extent, personal medical services should be rendered to the patient.
5. In so far as it would not, in the opinion of the doctor, be likely to cause serious damage to the physical or mental health of the patient to do so,

offer to discuss with the patient (or, where the patient is a child, the parent) the conclusions the doctor has drawn as a result of the consultation as to the state of the patient's health.

Patients not seen within three years

There is also a requirement to offer a similar health check to all patients aged 16–74 years on a general practitioner's list who have not been seen within the preceding three years. As part of such a health check the doctor (or nurse) is required to:

1. Where appropriate, seek details from the patient about his or her medical history and, as far as it may be relevant to the patient's medical history, about those of consanguineous family, in respect of:
   - illnesses, immunizations, allergies, hereditary diseases, medication, and health tests carried out for breast or cervical cancer;
   - social factors (including employment, housing, and family circumstances) that may affect his or her health;
   - factors of lifestyle (including diet, exercise, use of tobacco, consumption of alcohol, and misuse of drugs or solvents) that may affect his or her health; and
   - current state of health.
2. Offer to undertake a physical examination of the patient comprising:
   - the measurement of height, weight, and blood pressure; and
   - the taking of a urine sample for subsequent analysis to identify the presence of albumin and glucose.
3. Record, in the patient's medical records, findings arising out of the details supplied by, and any examination of, the patient.
4. Assess whether and, if so, in what manner and to what extent, personal medical services should be rendered to the patient.
5. In so far as it would not, in the opinion of the doctor, be likely to cause serious damage to the physical or mental health of the patient to do so, offer to discuss with the patient the conclusions the doctor has drawn as a result of the consultation as to the state of the patient's health.

Patients aged 75 years and over

For patients aged 75 years and over, the doctor is required to offer a home visit (either in person or by an appropriate member of the primary health care team) to assess the patient's health care needs. This assessment is to include any matter that appears to be affecting the patient's health including:

- sensory functions;
- mobility;
- mental condition;

- physical condition, including continence;
- social environment;
- use of medicines.

Again, the doctor is required to discuss with the patient the conclusions drawn, 'unless to do so would, in the opinion of the doctor, be likely to cause serious harm to the physical or mental health of the patient'.

Child health surveillance

It is not a requirement under the new contract for the general practitioner to provide child health surveillance health services as part of the obligation to be concerned with prevention of ill-health and promotion of good health, unless he or she has contracted specifically to do so by application for inclusion in the child health surveillance list, which in turn depends on appropriate qualifications and experience.

The service to which a qualified general practitioner is required to provide is for children under the age of 5 years, and includes:

1. The monitoring of the health, well-being, and physical, mental, and social development of the child with a view to detecting any deviations from normal development.
2. The examination of the child by or on behalf of the doctor on so many occasions and at such intervals as shall have been argued between the FHSA and the relevant health authority for the purposes of the provision of child health surveillance services generally in that district.

Contraceptive services

The new contract does not require a doctor to provide contraceptive services, as part of prevention of ill-health and promotion of good health, unless an undertaking has been given to provide such services by inclusion in the contraceptive list.

Target payments

As an incentive to general practitioners to achieve higher levels of cover for childhood immunization and for screening for cancer of the cervix, target payments have replaced the previous item of service fees. There are two levels of achievement. For childhood immunization, a higher level of payment is made to GPs who achieve 90 per cent coverage, and a lower level for those reaching 70 per cent. The differential in payment is 3:1. For screening for cervical cancer, the upper level is 80 per cent and the lower level 50 per cent, with the same differential applying, and the age-group concerned being 25–64 years.

The incorporation of health promotion and disease prevention

In the new terms of service of general practitioners, acknowledgement is made of a development that has been taking place for over a decade or more. Many practice teams have been gradually extending the services they provide; the expanding role of practice nurses has included many relevant activities. This expanded nursing role has been encouraged by re-imbursement of a substantial proportion (currently and in general 70 per cent) of nurses' salaries by the Department of Health. However, the imposition of 'cash limits' on such expenditure and the possibility of reduced re-imbursement will prejudice this development. The recognition of this development in the new contract ensures that it is an essential component of general practice, and no longer an optional service.

However, the specific requirement must be subject to critical review. In particular, the evidence for the effectiveness of health checks is limited. In recent years, there has been widespread adoption of nurse-conducted health checks, with nurses in a number of practices in each locality being trained and supported by facilitators. These health checks have generally been confined to the 35–64 years age-group on the premise that, by giving this age-group priority, the workload would not be overwhelming and the benefits likely to accrue would justify the effort involved. Moreover, for the same reasons, a five-yearly interval for review has been regarded as reasonable. Although there is evidence that such nurse-conducted health checks are successful in terms of population coverage and risk factor ascertainment, there is little evidence of their effectiveness in reducing morbidity and mortality. Research is currently being conducted which will throw some light on this issue. At present, a critical approach to this activity should be adopted because on present evidence, the requirement that those who have not consulted within a three-year period should have a 'health check' is difficult to justify.

Emphasis on 'health checks' may imply that the responsiblity for health and the prevention of disease is a matter for the individual and the health services alone. Although there is obvious scope for personal action, especially in relation to lifestyle, there are many constraints: a lack of information, advertising pressure, economic factors and the social environment all have important influences.

Health promotion clinics

A particular controversial aspect of the new general practice contract is the encouragement to set up 'health promotion clinics'. The *Statement of fees and allowances* payable to general medical practitioners from 1 April 1990 (para. 30) introduces a new fee for any health promotion 'clinic' that a doctor provides for patients on the practice list.

Eligibility is discretionary but to qualify for payment the following criteria must be satisfied:

1. Health promotion and illness prevention include initial surveillance of disease, disability and other health problems, and general advice and counselling on the maintenance of good health and well-being by the adoption of a healthy lifestyle. Clinics qualifying for payment include: well-man, well-woman, antismoking, alcohol control, diet, exercise counselling, stress management, heart disease prevention, and diabetes (this list is not exhaustive and clinics may cover more than one area).
2. Clinics held wholly or primarily for activities for which there is a separate payment (e.g. maternity services, cervical cytology, childhood immunization, child health surveillance, minor surgery, contraception) do not qualify.
3. A clinic 'session' must normally last at least one hour, must be advertised to patients in the local directory or practice leaflet, and be provided at separate appointments or through an 'open' appointment or group session. There must normally be at least 10 patients in any 'clinic'.

Provided these criteria are satisfied, a fee (in 1991: —45) may be claimed for each clinic; there appears to be no ceiling to the number of clinics for which payment may be made as long as the clinics are approved by the Family Health Services Authority (FHSA).

Clinics may be conducted by a general authority or by a suitably trained member of the practice team, and, in most cases, it is practice nurses who do the work.

Interpretation of the regulations by FHSAs has varied widely: some have applied the criteria rigidly; others have been flexible, accepting 'rolling' clinics, i.e. health promotion activities interspersed with other work as qualifying for payment. Some FHSAs have allowed the inclusion of opportunistic health promotion by general practitioners, in ordinary surgery consultation sessions (an interpretation that has been forbidden by the Department of Health because such activity is regarded as being remunerated within capitation fee payments).

Not surprisingly, therefore, 'health promotion clinics' are a contentious issue. It is widely accepted that prevention and health promotion are important aspects of primary health care, and this view is endorsed by their inclusion in the new terms of service. It is also generally acknowledged that the potential for these activities which arises from the opportunity created by patient-initiated 'illness consultations' is rarely explored. There are many reasons for this; a major reason is the brevity of such consultations. Consequently, the need for 'protected time' for health promotion and prevention bas been recognized, and the concept of a 'health promotion clinic' developed. However, the evidence of efficacy of such clinic-based interventions in terms of a benefit to health is lacking, but there is good evidence of efficacy of opportunistic health promotion as part of ordinary general practice advice–especially in achieving smoking cessation, but also in reducing alcohol consumption.

There seems to be a danger that opportunistic health promotion may be devalued and discouraged by the emphasis on health promotion clinics. Overall, net effect of health promotion clinics may be one of harm rather than benefit.

Postgraduate education

Finally, the new terms of service of general practitioners encourage continuing medical education, including education specifically in the field of prevention and health promotion.

A new allowance—the postgraduate education allowance (PGEA)—is paid to a general practitioner who has:

1. Attended 25 days of postgraduate education spread reasonably over the five years preceding the claim.
2. During that time attended at least two accredited courses in each of the following subject areas.
   - health promotion and prevention of illness;
   - disease management;
   - service management.

In 1991, the full allowance payable annually is £2025 and the establishment of this financial incentive appears to have been a major boost to postgraduate education.

Further reading

Department of Health (1989). *Terms of service for doctors in general practice.*

DHSS (1986). *Primary health care: an agenda for discussion.* HMSO, London.

DHSS (1987). *Promoting better health: the Government's programme for improving primary health care.* HMSO, London.

Health Departments of Great Britain (1989). *General practice in the National Health Service: the 1990 contract.*

Index